Praise for *Cancer Clinical Trials*

"...(the authors) decipher jargon and debunk myths, empowering patients to make more informed decisions. Setting the stage with the basics of cancer therapy and a brief history of clinical trials, the book moves quickly to the practical issues of finding a clinical trial and navigating the clinical trial system. I want all my patients (and all my trainees) to read this book."

—Kathy D. Miller, MD, Indiana University Melvin and Bren Simon Cancer Center, Indianapolis

". . . fills the need for a thorough yet plain-language guide explaining the benefits (and also the risks) of clinical trial participation. . . a valuable and up-to-date overview of cancer treatment, including all the major modalities: surgery, radiation, chemotherapy, the newer targeted therapies, and immunotherapy. . . also considers important practical issues such as costs, insurance coverage, regulatory oversight, and the use of placebos . . . a welcome addition to the literature available to cancer patients who want to explore all practical options for ensuring that they get the best therapy possible, and for accelerating research toward new cancer cures."

—David Josephy, President, GIST Sarcoma Life Raft Group Canada

". . . valuable for patients and their family members and friends facing a battle with cancer, as (the book) can inform and empower people to seek the best care available. In a straightforward manner, it not only outlines what cancer is and how treatment is approached now and will be in the future, it shares how treatments are moved forward through experimentation in clinical trials. It provides helpful suggestions on how to find and benefit from such trials and address challenges one might have in the search. Dialog and communication between patient and doctor is so essential, this book can inform patients and promotes informed discussion and involvement."

—Thomas N. Kirk, President/CEO, Us TOO International Prostate Cancer Education and Support Network

"Being diagnosed with cancer can be a frightening experience that leaves one lost in a strange landscape of unfamiliar tests, big words, and bigger choices. Drs. Beer and Axmaker provide a road map that not only guides the reader through the complex twists and turns of cancer diagnosis and treatment, but empowers patients and family members to ask informed questions and make informed decisions about cancer clinical trials...

Every cancer patient interested in a clinical trial should understand the key concepts outlined in this book. The authors explain complicated technical terms and procedures in simple, clear language and take away some of the anxiety associated with the unknown."

—James L. Gulley, MD, PhD, FACP, Director, Clinical Trials Group, National Cancer Institute

"... a comprehensive and highly accessible resource for understanding modern cancer therapeutics. It explains beautifully the complex process of designing, undertaking, and interpreting clinical trials in cancer. It does so in the wider context of understanding what elements are addressed in deciding what the best treatment is for any particular patient. Anyone faced with the diagnosis of cancer and hoping to understand how to navigate treatment in our modern age will find this book extremely valuable. I also feel this book should be read by medical and nursing students as a first rate introduction in the basics of both clinical trials and cancer therapeutics."

—Joseph T. Ruggiero, MD, Medical Director, Solid Tumor Oncology Practice, Weill Cornell Medical College, New York

"... a powerful, practical, and accessible account of how to navigate cancer clinical trials. In addition to providing a detailed assessment of the various risks and benefits associated with participation in cancer clinical trials as well as insight into how clinical trials are designed and run, the book features "bottom line" sections at the end of each chapter that succinctly summarize the important take-away issues that patients should consider... For anyone affected by cancer such as patients, health professionals, families, caregivers, and loved ones, (this book) should be required reading."

—Jonathan W. Simons, MD, President and CEO, David H. Koch Chair of the Prostate Cancer Foundation

". . . (a) well-balanced explanation on every aspect of clinical trials . . . Written in plain, lay-people's language, despite its content being highly scientific and technical. . ."

—Seiichi Ariga, PhD, University chaplain (retired)

". . . a thoughtful, easy-to-read guide to demystify the clinical trials process, explain the risks and benefits, and educate patients about their role in this critically important endeavor. . . In a day and age when increasing pressure is placed on the patient to take control of his or her medical care, this guide provides understandable answers to potential trial participants' most frequently asked questions, while debunking myths and providing pointers to additional sources of information. . . a guide that makes it possible for patients to put their best foot forward when making important treatment decisions."

—Skip Lockwood, President and CEO,
ZERO—The Project to End Prostate Cancer

". . . brilliant in the easy way (this book) introduces patients to the pros and cons of participating in those much-needed studies. . . informs patients about how to find appropriate trials to participate in and what to expect from that experience. . . (an) easily accessible introduction to the breadth of treatments both currently available and in development . . . for patients who truly want others to benefit from their experience—this is *the book*. . ."

—Richard Wassersug, PhD, prostate cancer patient;
researcher, Dept. of Urologic Sciences, University of British Columbia,
Vancouver, British Columbia, Canada

"*Cancer Clinical Trials* is a treasure. The cover states the book contains 'everything you need to know about clinical trials,' and that understates the case; it has everything and more! The book is clearly written and quite understandable. It lists the nuts and bolts behind how trials are done, why patients might (and should!) participate, and what they should ask their doctor, before, during, and after, deciding and participating in a study. Ethical issues are covered delicately but appropriately. I cannot imagine a more useful book for anyone touched by cancer or who knows someone thinking about options."

—Charles D. Blanke, MD, FACP, FRCPC, Vice President,
Systemic Therapy, British Columbia Cancer Agency;
Professor and Head, Division of Medical Oncology,
University of British Columbia

"This book should be required reading for cancer patients and their family members for so many reasons. It not only discusses the current effective options, but also covers the potential breakthrough treatments in cancer that are happening right now, and it even provides expert guidance on the maze of health insurance issues that many cancer patients and their health care professionals deal with today. Best of all, this book is not filled with confusing medical jargon, but rather provides an easy-to-understand guide to help you in the decision making process."

—Mark A. Moyad, MD, MPH, Department of Urology, University of Michigan Medical Center, Ann Arbor

"... *Cancer Clinical Trials* is a valuable tool to (improving survival rate)... by clearing up misconceptions about cancer clinical trials, and aiding patients as they decide about participation in cancer clinical trials. This book is both comprehensive and easy to use, with direct questions asked and answered, misconceptions you may encounter highlighted, and samples of practical items such as billing schedules and insurance letters provided. In the end, readers are invited to join the authors, and advocates like myself, into this cancer fighting community."

—Brandon Hayes-Lattin, MD, Senior Medical Advisor, LIVESTRONG; Medical Director, Adolescent and Young Adult Oncology Program, Knight Cancer Institute, Portland, OR

"Clinical trials are a critical component of our cancer care delivery system, and they will unlock new therapies that will benefit many individuals and families in the future. (This) new book helps educate us all as to the complexity and inner workings of these trials."

—Doug Ulman, President/CEO, LIVESTRONG, The Lance Armstrong Foundation

Cancer Clinical Trials

A Commonsense Guide to Experimental Cancer Therapies and Clinical Trials

Tomasz M. Beer, MD
and
Larry W. Axmaker, EdD

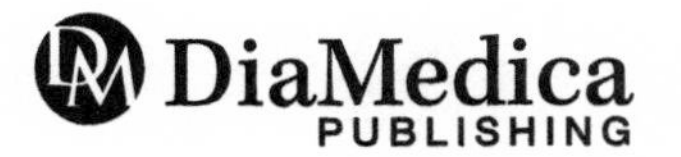

DiaMedica Publishing, 150 East 61st Street, New York, NY 10065

Visit our website at www.diamedicapub.com

ISBN: 978-0-9823219-7-3 (print)
ISBN: 978-1-936832-17-0 (e-book)

Library of Congress Cataloging-in-Publication Data is available from the publisher.

DiaMedica titles are available for bulk purchase, special promotions, and premiums. For more information please contact the publisher through the publisher's website: www.diamedicapub.com.

Disclaimer:
The content in this book is not intended as a substitute for medical or professional counseling and advice. The reader is encouraged to consult his or her physicians and therapists on all health matters, especially symptoms that may require professional diagnosis and/or medical attention.

Book design: TypeWriting
Cover design: Gopa & Ted2
Editors: Jessica Bryan and Joann Woy

The authors of this book will be pleased to respond to your questions and comments on their blog at: www.cancer-clinical-trials.com.

Dedication

To Angie, and to Maria and Sofia

—Tom

To Carol, for 50 years of love, patience, and support

—Larry

Acknowledgments

We gratefully acknowledge the extensive and invaluable comments of Kristi Eilers. We also gratefully acknowledge the invaluable feedback we received from Sandra Wendel, Mandy Burns, David Josephy, Cynthia Chauhan, and members of the Patient Advocates Committee of the Alliance for Clinical Trials in Oncology.

We also appreciate the efforts of the staff at DiaMedica, including Dr. Diana M. Schneider, Patty Wallenburg, Jessica Bryan, and Joann Woy.

Tom is thankful for the support of his co-workers at Oregon Health & Science University's Knight Cancer Institute, whose hard work made his sabbatical and this book possible.

Larry is grateful for the support of his family and friends, and for the medical advances that have kept his cancer under control for many years. Larry also extends his gratitude to Tom for inviting him to collaborate on this project.

About the Authors

Tomasz M. Beer, MD, is a medical oncologist (cancer specialist). He leads a research and clinical trial program at Oregon Health & Science University Knight Cancer Institute in Portland, Oregon. Dr. Beer has dedicated his professional life to improving the care of cancer patients through the development of new and better treatments. He has been directly involved in over 100 clinical trials, and he has treated hundreds of cancer patients who chose investigational therapy, as well as thousands who did not.

Dr. Beer has led trials at all phases, from trials that study a medication previously tested only in animals and test it for the first time in human beings, to large international trials that compare treatments to each other and that, if successful, change the standard of cancer care.

In many ways, he has seen all sides of clinical trials. He has been involved in studies that produced more effective treatments and that are now routinely used, and he has also conducted studies that failed to help treat cancer. He has seen both unexpected successes and unexpected side effects.

Dr. Beer is deeply dedicated to cancer research. He believes that research is the best way forward, but he is also acutely aware of the blind alleys and pitfalls that can mar some clinical trials. It is his hope that this book will help you enter into the often mysterious world of clinical trials armed with information and well prepared for the decisions you will be called upon to make.

Larry W. Axmaker, EdD, is a retired psychologist, teacher, and writer. He has prostate cancer and has participated in several clinical trials. Dr. Axmaker recently published a book about prostate cancer entitled *Real Men Get Prostate Cancer Too*, which chronicles his sometimes serious, sometimes humorous journey with cancer.

Dr. Axmaker worked as a clinical psychologist and university instructor in psychology for many years, and has helped train psychologists, social workers, and counselors. He is an award-winning writer in the health and medicine field, where he worked for more than a dozen years exploring the process and progress of medical research and its benefits. Dr. Axmaker would like to see more cancer clinical trials conducted and better treatments developed—to help himself *and* others, perhaps including *you*.

Contents

Preface

THIS BOOK WAS DESIGNED to help people with cancer decide if a clinical trial is a good option for their particular situations, to choose a clinical trial that might be of benefit for their specific situations, and to navigate through the clinical trial process. It will provide you with a basic understanding of clinical trials and the various types of trials, as well as lists of questions to ask, things to look for, things to watch out for, places to look, and ways to find the right person to answer your questions. The book will help you learn why you might want to consider participating in clinical trials, and how to make an educated and beneficial decision.

Unlike most books about clinical trials—which are written for the professionals who run them—we only discuss the technical details and knowledge that can help people with cancer and their families consider what role clinical trials might play in their personal cancer care.

Cancer is treated in many different ways, including surgery, radiation therapy, medications (chemotherapy and many other types of medications), complementary methods, exercise, diet, and more. We generally refer to the various medications used to treat cancer as "medical therapy." Virtually all of these treatments are available because they were developed through research. Although there are many types of treatment and many different cancers, we have divided this complex world into two broad categories: *standard care* (regular, approved treatment by your doctor and medical team) and *experimental* or *investigational therapy* (in which you participate in a clinical trial).

A Quick Word About Experimental Therapy

- *Experimental therapy* and *investigational therapy* are interchangeable terms. They mean that the therapy is still being developed, evaluated, or refined, and it has not yet been fully established. In other words, the Food and Drug Administration (FDA)—the national regulatory agency in the United States—has not approved it as a standard prescribed treatment, and it is not recognized as such by the medical community.
- Experimental therapy is always given to patients as part of a *clinical trial*, the structure within which experimental therapy is provided. It is the recipe, the program, the schedule, and the rulebook that defines the *who*, the *how*, and the *when* of experimental therapy. In this book, we sometimes refer to "experimental or investigational therapy," while at other times we use the words "clinical trial." In general, we are writing about the same thing.

If you are reading this book, you probably fall into one of these groups:

- You have cancer and are seeking *something more*. In this case, a clinical trial might be just what you are looking for; or
- You know someone who could use the information to make an important choice in his or her life.

We join together as doctor and patient, as researcher and clinical trial participant, as medical health professional and mental health professional, and as two human beings dedicated to giving you a clear, comprehensive, and unvarnished guide to experimental cancer therapy. We hope you will learn everything you need to know about the potential promises and perils of cancer clinical trials.

Tomasz M. Beer, MD and Larry W. Axmaker, EdD
January 2012

Introduction

ALL OF THE *STANDARD* CANCER THERAPIES currently available were developed in clinical trials. Clinical trials are experiments—highly organized and complex experiments that test new therapies in volunteers who have the specific type of cancer being evaluated in the trial.

Thousands of experimental cancer drugs and treatments exist that have not yet been tested in humans. One of the most important roadblocks to progress against cancer is that many clinical trials fail to attract enough participants. Fewer than 5 percent of adults with cancer ever participate in a clinical trial, and *nearly one in three* clinical trials fail to enroll a single participant. There are, of course, other barriers to progress, including limited investment in research, the biologic complexity of cancer, challenges in developing effective and safe drugs that shut down some of cancer's growth mechanisms, and the potential for unpleasant side effects from promising new drugs. New ideas that already exist may hold answers to the challenges that stand in the way of successful cancer treatment, but they cannot result in improvements in treatment until they are evaluated in a clinical trial.

This is true even at major cancer centers. Depending on whose numbers you trust, between 22 and 60 percent of phase III clinical trials fail to attract enough participants to finish the job, even when they are conducted at dozens of centers. These trials should be testing the best new ideas against the current gold standard treatment and answering the important questions. Does this matter to you? Absolutely!

Progress in treating cancer in children has been more rapid than advances in treatments for adults with cancer. Children with cancer are often treated at academic medical centers that focus on research. As a result, children have largely been treated as part of clinical trials. According to the National Cancer Institute (NCI), 80 percent of children are still alive 5 years after receiving a diagnosis of cancer. In the mid-1970s, this figure was 62 percent. Pediatric cancer research has reduced the death rate from children's cancers from nearly 40 percent to about 20 percent, eliminating nearly half of the cancer deaths that were occurring 30 years ago! Between 55 and 65 percent of children under the age of 14 receive their treatment as part of a clinical trial. This is a staggering rate of participation. For children, a clinical trial *is* the standard of care.

Children, of course, might have some advantages other than clinical trial participation to explain the striking improvements in outcomes. Their bodies are more resilient and better able to recover from cancer therapies. Their cancers are biologically different and—in some cases—perhaps easier to cure or treat. But one message is clear: the secrets to success in treating pediatric cancers have been unlocked through clinical trials.

By now, you may be thinking that we are unabashed clinical trial enthusiasts—and we are, when we think about it from the perspective of society. There is no question that the cancer patients of tomorrow will benefit from successful clinical trials being conducted today. We are also enthusiastic when we think about it from the perspective of individuals with cancer. We believe that a clinical trial may be the best choice for many people at some point in the course of a battle with cancer.

We also know that clinical trials are not for everyone. Not all clinical trials are successful. Not all participants in a successful clinical trial will benefit equally, and some may receive no benefit at all or even experience some harm.

So, we are going to take you on a journey into the world of clinical trials, one that will inform and support your personal decisions—whatever they may turn out to be. Where confusion and uncertainty exist, we will "pop the hood and peek underneath." We won't try to sell you on clinical trials. We will "tell it like it is" and give you tools to help you decide what to do.

Should you decide to pursue participation in a clinical trial, we will also provide the information you need to navigate your way through the process.

How Should You Use This Book?

This guide to investigational therapies for cancer will introduce you to the history of clinical trials and their general structure, give you an overview of the types of new treatments that are being tested, discuss the details of how clinical trials work, and tell you what the experience of being a participant can be like.

We will also focus on specific practical issues that you may face: how to find a clinical trial that makes sense for you, how to interact with your health insurance carrier, how to approach selecting a clinical trial, and what to do while you are a participant. And finally, we provide a glimpse into the future of clinical trials, a guide to cancer drugs, and a glossary of technical terms you need to know.

We invite you to use this book in whatever way serves you best. You may want to read it cover to cover, or you may wish to jump to those chapters that cover specific issues that you are facing right now. Chances are you will find a few "pearls of wisdom," even if you are already familiar with the core concepts.

An Overview of Core Concepts in Clinical Trials

To help orient you to the material that will be covered in this book, here is a summary of the key topics that we will discuss in detail in subsequent chapters.

What *Is* Cancer and How Is It Treated?

Modern cancer treatments have their basis in the nature of the cancer cell. Understanding what we know about the unique nature of cancer cells and tumors, plus the three basic approaches to cancer care—surgery, medical therapy (medications), and radiation therapy—provides the background you will need to make a decision about whether a clinical trial might be right for you and how you can evaluate all of your available options.

What Is a Clinical Trial and Why Might You Want to Consider Joining One?

You may be considering a clinical trial because no appropriate standard therapy is available; the current standard leaves room for improvement; or because you don't need treatment right away because your cancer is slow-growing and you would like to try something new.

Many new ideas are being evaluated in clinical trials today, for a broad variety of cancers. Chemotherapy and hormonal therapy have been around for a long time, but these treatments are still being improved. In addition, many new types of cancer drugs are being developed, including:

- Drugs designed to stimulate the immune system to fight cancer
- Artificial antibodies that target key components of cancer
- Custom-made chemicals that bind to and disable various drivers of cancer growth and cancer survival
- Drugs designed to turn on and off specific genes that may be responsible for cancer growth and for cancer's ability to spread throughout the human body

Innovation is not limited to medications. Clinical trials are also examining new approaches and new technologies in surgery, radiation therapy, and other areas of cancer treatment.

How Are Clinical Trials Designed and Run?

Clinical Trials Are Divided Into Phases

There are many kinds of clinical trials, but they are generally organized into a series of *phases*:

- Phase I studies are small, and their goal is to determine the optimal dose of a drug, or combination of drugs, that can be given safely. This does not mean entirely free of side effects, just an acceptable or manageable level of side effects.
- Phase II studies are also relatively small and may involve anywhere between 30 and several hundred patients. They are the first studies designed to test how effective a new treatment is against cancer.
- Phase III studies are large and may involve thousands of participants. They compare the most promising new treatments to the current standard.
- Phase IV studies usually collect more safety and effectiveness information on new therapies after the U.S. Food and Drug Administration has approved them.

When all goes well, a new treatment progresses through all these phases and becomes a new standard of care—meaning it is considered the best available treatment for a particular type of cancer. Many treatments don't make it through this process and are found to be either too toxic (in phase I studies) or not effective enough (in phase II or phase III studies). Unfortunately, it is impossible to pick the winners ahead of time, and there are no guarantees in the process.

Some Clinical Trials Are Randomized and Often Blinded

In phase I and many phase II studies, all patients receive the same treatment. Randomized trials are then used to compare the new treatment being studied to the current best standard treatments. *Randomization* ensures that the two groups of patients being compared to one another in a clinical trial—those getting the new treatment and those getting the established one or a *placebo*—are as similar to each other as possible. This gives researchers confidence that if a difference is found between the two groups, then it was the treatment that made the difference. Placebos are never used as a substitute for an effective and established treatment. They can be added to an effective treatment in a study that offers the current standard treatment to all participants. Placebos are used alone only when the standard approach would be to monitor the cancer without treatment.

Randomized studies are often *blinded*. This means that you and your doctor won't know which of the two treatments you are receiving. Blinding often involves a placebo—an inactive drug that looks like the real one. Blinding is done to further reduce *bias* that might creep into a study. Biases can deceive us into thinking that one treatment is better than another, when the difference is actually due to patients and doctors behaving differently during different treatments.

How Can I Choose a Trial That's Right for *Me*?

Deciding whether to participate in a clinical trial at all, and choosing one that you are comfortable with, can be difficult. Your cancer diagnosis may be new and fresh in your mind. Just dealing with that can be enormously taxing. Clinical trials add complexity and create additional uncertainty. You will likely need plenty of advice and support as you navigate these challenging waters. Your doctor and possibly another physician who can offer a second opinion, your family, friends, spiritual advisors, and support groups of fellow cancer survivors can all provide the support you need to make these choices and move forward. Clinical trials can offer you additional hope through the knowledge that you may have more options than you originally thought. You will also be helping researchers find better treatments, not just for the next generation, but hopefully for you, too.

Once you have decided that you want to consider participating in a clinical trial, finding one that is a good match can be quite a challenge.

If your doctor is affiliated with a medical center that conducts multiple research studies, it may be as simple as discussing your options with him. In Chapter 6, we discuss the best ways to search for trials online, including, most importantly, the National Cancer Institute's website: www.cancer.gov. Knowing the type and stage of your cancer, the treatments you have received so far, your general health, the types of studies you are interested in, and how far you are willing to travel for treatment can help you narrow the search to a manageable number of options.

Who Is Looking Out for You and What Are the Costs of Participating?

Your Legal and Medical Rights If You Participate in a Trial

Clinical trials are carefully monitored for safety. Here, we will review the structure of a trial and the features that will be in place for your protection.

What Are the Costs of Participating in a Clinical Trial?

The potential cost of participating in clinical trials is a frequent concern for many people with cancer. The answer is not simple, but often the news is favorable. In general, clinical trials that test treatments for cancer provide the new drug being investigated free of charge, and they also cover procedures that are being done solely for research purposes. The things that routinely happen in the course of cancer care—such as physician visits, routine lab tests, and scans—are generally billed to you and your health insurance provider. Recognizing that improvement in cancer care is a good thing for all of us, most insurers are willing to cover these costs. But that is not always the case. Medicare covers the costs in the United States, with some restrictions. The majority of states have passed laws requiring that state-regulated health plans also cover such costs. You should check with your insurance company and, if required, get preapproval for coverage, so that you can participate in a clinical trial with peace of mind.

Much of this book describes fundamental principles of clinical trials, and these apply all over the world. Some parts of the book are focused on the United States. This is especially true of Chapter 8, in which we discuss health insurance and costs of clinical care during a clinical trials. Other countries' health insurance systems differ widely in how they approach clinical trials. If you are thinking about participating in a clinical trial outside of the United States, please check with your health insurance provider and research team about any costs.

Clinical trials are increasingly international, and often the same clinical trials are open in many countries at once. As a result, apart from insurance and legal protections that differ somewhat from country to country, the information in the book should be worthwhile regardless of where you live.

What Can I Expect During a Clinical Trial?

Once you are a part of a clinical trial, you can expect certain things from your research and care team. They will have some expectations of you, too. Most importantly, you should expect expert and attentive care—sometimes more attention than you are accustomed to. You should expect open, honest, and complete communication. All of your questions should be answered, and all your concerns addressed. You can't expect that the treatment will always work, or that it will be free of side effects. But you *can* expect that your cancer will be closely monitored, so that your treatment can be stopped or changed if it's not working. Any side effects will also be closely followed, and hopefully adjustments can be made to reduce or eliminate them.

You will retain the right to withdraw from the study at any time, but you should discuss your concerns with your research team and your doctor first. You may learn that your difficulties can be addressed. If not, you will need their advice and support to discontinue therapy in an orderly fashion and transition to some other cancer treatment in a safe and timely manner.

The most important thing the research team will expect from you is open, honest, and timely communication. They want and need to know how you are doing, and they need to know about any side effects promptly. It is important for your safety that you inform your research team about any side effects. The team will also expect you to take your commitment to the study seriously. There may be more visits, more tests, and more surveys than you are used to. This can be a hardship, or at the very least quite time-consuming, but all of it is important if the study is to succeed.

What Cancer Treatments Are Currently Available?

This section will provide you with the information you need to understand the range of treatments now in existence, emphasizing chemotherapy and newer approaches such as targeted therapy.

Misconceptions About Clinical Trials

Misconceptions about clinical trials are common. Misunderstandings about all aspects of clinical trials, from purpose and key design features to the likelihood of success, and to costs and expectations, can lead to disappointment. Excessive pessimism or optimism about your prospects, whether with standard or experimental treatment, can lead to flawed decisions about your treatment. Throughout this book, we provide examples of the common misconceptions we have encountered and some key information to help you avoid or overcome them. Look for the "A Misconception You May Encounter" sections that appear in several chapters.

Future Trends in Clinical Trials

We expect future clinical trials to become more focused on *personalizing therapy*. Most of today's therapies are tested in large groups of patients with the same cancer. Such studies try to find an overall benefit for the entire group of patients. Unfortunately, they are not able to determine in advance which individual patients will benefit the most or the least. Research is changing from the "one size fits all" approach—involving trial-and-error therapy in each patient—to a much more individualized approach. Sophisticated analyses of each cancer and each patient increasingly enable us to select the right therapy for each patient the first time. Some of the newest cancer drugs are being approved together with specific tests that enable physicians to determine if a particular patient is likely to benefit from treatment. In the clinical trials of the future, we will look at *collections of individuals*, each of whom receives a uniquely designed treatment, rather than at *groups* whose members are all treated the same.

Part I

Cancer and Cancer Treatment Basics

1

What Is Cancer and How Is It Treated?

Treating cancer is much more complicated than researchers believed possible even a few decades ago. The newest research is helping us understand what causes cancer, and this, in turn, is leading to more effective treatments. Before we discuss cancer therapy and clinical trials, it would be helpful to understand a bit about what cancer *is.*

What Is Cancer?

Some important similarities exist between cancer and common infectious diseases, particularly chronic infections, such as tuberculosis. Like cancer, infections can invade the human body, grow out of control, and destroy normal cells. However, organisms that invade our bodies from the outside cause infections. The fact that these invaders are different from us biologically is what makes many effective treatments possible. *Antibiotics* are poisonous to bacteria but relatively safe for us. They are designed to attack processes or molecules that are important for the growth of bacteria but that don't normally exist in the healthy human body. Bacteria are different enough from our own cells that we can safely kill them without harming ourselves.

Cancer, however, starts and grows from *within* our bodies. A human body develops from a single fertilized egg, which divides and develops the unique cell types that make up the organs of our bodies. When all is well, these cells behave as they should and die when their work is done. Most cells grow and divide before they die. The cells of most organs in the body divide and multiply more or less frequently. The skin cells and the cells of our gastrointestinal tract regularly replace themselves, while cells in other organs are replaced less frequently. These processes must happen correctly for our body to function as it should. Things wouldn't work very well, for example, if our skin cells grew but never died—the term "thick skin" would take on a whole new meaning! Cancers are often divided into *solid tumors*, which originate from the organs of the body and begin as local growths or lumps that later spread, and *liquid tumors*, cancers of the blood and bone marrow cells that often circulate in the blood stream.

Cancer is caused by a disruption of this healthy natural state. A classic article by Douglas Hanahan and Robert A. Weinberg, "The Hallmarks of Cancer," captures the basics of the disease. They described six primary characteristics (hallmarks) of cancer. Their work has been widely accepted, and it has changed the thinking of researchers about how to develop anticancer treatments.

The Six Hallmarks of Cancer

Six main features are considered to be the *hallmarks* of the disease we call cancer:

- The ability of cells to grow without requiring a growth signal from the rest of the body to do so. Cancer cells have their own, self-sufficient *growth engine* that is not subject to the needs of the body as a whole.
- Resistance to natural anti-growth instructions. Cancers do not respond to the normal controls that the body places on growth; as a result, they reproduce indiscriminately.

- The ability to invade and spread throughout the body.
- The ability to continue dividing and growing without end. In a manner of speaking, cancer cells are immortal. While this hallmark has much in common with the first two, the ability to grow without growth signals and resist normal breaks could be a temporary condition, but in cancer it is not. It is a permanent defect that is responsible for the relentless nature of cancer.
- Cancer has the ability to recruit cells that make up the vascular system in order to develop its own blood supply, thereby ensuring a flow of nutrients to support the cancer's growth.
- The ability to evade natural death.

Cancer can therefore be defined as a disease of unchecked, abnormal growth that attracts its own nourishment, spreads, and has the ability to evade death. Normal cells are not supposed to do *any* of these things. To grow and cause us harm, cancer has to do *all* of them. It has to have all six characteristics, each of which is caused by multiple defects in the cell's function. These defects are the targets of many cancer treatments. As we learn more about which defects lead to each of these hallmarks in each type of cancer—different cancers are caused by different kinds of defects—we will become better at developing and designing cancer drugs and treatments.

Cancer is a disease of unchecked, abnormal growth that attracts its own nourishment, spreads, and has the ability to evade death.

The Three Mainstays of Cancer Treatment

The three main cancer treatments currently in use are: surgery, radiation, and the broad category of *medical therapy* or medications. The medications category includes much more than just chemotherapy, as we will discuss later in this chapter. All three of these treatment types are continually being improved through research, both in the laboratory and in clinical trials. If you are contemplating becoming a part of a clinical trial, it is likely that an innovation in one of these three principal treatments will be involved. It is impossible to account for every area of active research, so what follows are the most common.

Surgery

Surgery is the oldest treatment for cancer. Simply put, the basic goal of surgery is to remove the cancer. There are four important areas in which surgery has improved in recent years, and where research is now focused: new technology, less surgery, more precise surgery, and the combination of surgery with other treatments.

New Technology

A major improvement in surgery has been to use new technologies to make the surgical experience both less invasive and less extensive. One example is laparoscopic surgery, which involves the use of highly specialized instruments to perform complex surgical procedures through small incisions. Many major operations that, in the past, required a large surgical opening can now be performed through much smaller ones. The result is less pain and faster recovery. These techniques are increasingly being used in cancer surgery. Some operations even use a robotic assistant to facilitate laparoscopic surgeries. You may encounter clinical studies designed to test these new surgical approaches or to compare one approach to another.

There are also new technologies that do not use a traditional surgical knife (scalpel). Focused ultrasound (high-intensity sound waves that we cannot hear), focused radio waves, freezing therapy (cryotherapy), and even injections of alcohol and other substances are examples of techniques that can sometimes be used to shrink or even eliminate a tumor. These technologies are also being improved through research, and they are sometimes compared against conventional surgery in clinical trials.

Less Surgery

Early cancer surgeons often used extensive surgery to take no chances—removing too much rather than too little. While these approaches were often effective, they could be quite disfiguring as well. Over the last century, surgeons have sought to maintain high cure rates while keeping the surgery as limited as possible. Major strides have been made in this area.

For example, breast cancer surgery began as a procedure that removed not just the breast, but also a considerable portion of the chest wall muscles. Research led first to the development of modern mastectomy—removal of the breast but not major muscles. More recently, even less invasive approaches have become common. *Lumpectomies*, for example, remove only the tumor tissue and spare the unaffected portions of the breast.

Research in this area continues to focus on the minimum surgery necessary to do the job against cancer. In some cases, less extensive surgery is made possible by combining surgery with other cancer treatments, such as radiation and/or medications.

More Precise Surgery

An improved understanding of human anatomy and how cancer spreads has led to more successful removal of cancer and fewer side effects from treatment. You might think that we have already learned just about all there is to know about these things, especially human anatomy, but there are subtle details we have learned only recently, and we're still learning more. For example, the precise location of the nerves responsible for male sexual function and how they can be spared during prostate surgery is a relatively recent advance. The precise patterns by which cancers spread are still being discovered, as the result of better medical imaging and meticulous research by surgeons. This knowledge about patterns of cancer spread is important, for example, in determining which lymph nodes need to be removed in addition to the primary tumor.

Surgery in Combination with Other Treatments

Whether to improve overall cure rates or reduce the extent of the surgery needed to successfully remove tumors, cancer care increasingly involves multiple treatment types given together. Surgery is increasingly accompanied by anticancer medications, radiation therapy, or both. These can be given before or after surgery, depending on the type of cancer.

Radiation Therapy

Radiation damages cancer cells, causing them to die, while at the same time attempting to spare normal human tissue. This process is less than perfect, although it is dramatically better than it used to be. When normal tissues are exposed to radiation, the resulting damage—which may be temporary or permanent—can lead to side effects. It is not surprising that radiation research is focused on increasing the precision of radiation delivery. The goal is to maximize the dose of radiation delivered to damage and kill the tumor, while minimizing the dose delivered to normal tissue. Some of the ways research is advancing these goals include new technologies to increase the precision of radiation, the development of new types of radiation, and the combination of radiation with other therapies.

New Technologies for More Precise Targeting of Radiation

We have come a long way from just exposing the general area of the tumor to a radiation beam. Today, sophisticated computer programs control dozens, if not hundreds, of beams that all cross precisely within the tumor tissue. Research to refine the targeting of these beams continues. One example of an active area of investigation is implanting "beacons" into the tumor to serve as targets. These beacons allow the radiation beam to follow the tumor even if it moves slightly due to normal breathing, normal movements of the bowels, or inadvertent movements by the patient.

New Types of Radiation

Proton beam radiation is an example of a new form of radiation. Protons are actually tiny charged particles found in the nuclei of atoms. The smallest atom—hydrogen—consists of one proton and one electron. Proton therapy showers the cancer with tiny particles that are accelerated to high speeds. Protons are the only type of new particle radiation therapy now available for routine use, but others are being developed. Several centers, principally outside of the United States, are experimenting with carbon ions, another type of charged particles. Charged particle therapy may offer a way to deliver more radiation to the tumor with less damage to surrounding tissues. Research will be necessary to prove this, of course. Other approaches include using radioactive molecules that are attached to antibodies specific for the tumor tissue, and therefore transported through the bloodstream to areas invaded by tumor cells.

Combination Therapies

Medications taken before or during radiation can sensitize cancer to radiation. Such approaches may allow lower doses of radiation to be just as effective as higher ones, without some of the risks and side effects. They may also improve the effectiveness of radiation delivered at standard doses.

Medical Therapy (Medications)

When we think about clinical trials in cancer, we most often think about studies that involve new drugs. Most of this book focuses on studies of new cancer drugs, because a great deal of effort is under way in this area, and a large number of cancer drugs are now in clinical trials. To help you make sense of them, here are the broad categories:

Chemotherapy

Chemotherapy can be considered the "granddaddy" of all cancer drug treatments. Dr. Sidney Farber first conceived this approach in 1948. He recognized that *folate*, a common B vitamin, is needed by leukemia cells to grow. He then demonstrated that drugs that blocked folate could, for a time, markedly reduce the number of leukemic cells in the blood of leukemia patients. Chemotherapy became a catch-all name for a large number of cancer drugs that work through a variety of mechanisms. Many chemotherapy drugs are given as an intravenous infusion into the vein, but some chemotherapy drugs are taken in pill form.

Chemotherapy has a bit of a bad reputation because many of these drugs damage not only cancer cells, but also cells in other organs of the body. This is what causes chemotherapy's well-known unpleasant side effects, such as hair loss and nausea. One reason for side effects is that, in order to have the desired effect on cancer cells, the drugs often have to be given at high doses that also affect healthy cells.

Chemotherapy can be considered the "granddaddy" of all cancer drug treatments.

Although most modern clinical trials involve studies of newer, more targeted, and more selective drugs, you may still encounter chemotherapy drugs that have been available for many years. There are good reasons for this. For example, some of the newer targeted drugs work best in combination with standard chemotherapy. Chemotherapy drugs are still being improved. For some cancers, they offer reliable cures, and for many cancers, they will continue to play a major role in the future.

Hormonal Therapy

Some cancers—breast and prostate cancers in particular—are dependent on *sex hormones*, such as estrogen and testosterone. These cancers can often be treated by lowering overall hormone levels or by blocking cancer cells' access to hormones. Hormonal therapy has been available for more than 60 years. However, recent discoveries have shown that today's drugs do not fully suppress hormonal activity. Newer and more powerful hormone blockers are being developed and tested. They generally focus either on reducing the production of hormones in the body or on blocking hormone *receptors*, the key entry portals for hormones into the cells. While some hormonal drugs must be injected into the muscle or under the skin, many are available in pill form. Hormonal drugs are on the "short list" of drugs that have also been shown to reduce the risk of developing cancer.

Immunologic Therapy

The immune system appears to play a major role in detecting abnormal cancer cells. This is a difficult task because cancer cells evolve from normal cells and often are not sufficiently different from normal cells for the immune system to identify and destroy them. We don't actually know much about the success of the immune system in detecting and destroying cancer cells, but we think that cancers are constantly being eliminated or controlled before they can become major tumors. We don't know how frequently this happens, because these abnormal cells or tiny cancers are never detected in the first place. It's a bit like the CIA—when the immune system succeeds, you never know about it. We *do* know that the immune system can sometimes eliminate even advanced cancers. We see this when drugs that stimulate the immune system eliminate advanced kidney cancer or melanoma.

Unfortunately, the immune-stimulating drugs currently available rarely succeed; they don't help most patients at all. Why these treatments work for some people but not others is one of the pressing mysteries in current cancer research. However, the occasional successes prove that the immune system *can* destroy cancer. Many researchers are motivated to find more and better ways to help our immune systems do this.

A number of approaches to stimulate immune function are now being studied in clinical trials. These can generally be divided into two categories: cancer vaccines and immune system–stimulating drugs. Vaccines rely on finding unique cancer *antigens*—proteins that are only present on cancer cells and absent in normal cells, and that can be recognized by the immune system—and giving them to the patient in combination with drugs that stimulate immune recognition and action.

Immune system–activating drugs are not tumor-specific, like vaccines, but instead stimulate the immune system in a general way and rely on the enhanced immune system to detect cancer and attack it.

Both approaches can have positive effects, and a combination of the two may be a promising strategy. A lot more work needs to be done to better understand the immune system and how to stimulate it to destroy cancers.

Monoclonal Antibodies

Antibodies are made by our natural immune system to fight infections. We can make artificial antibodies against almost anything, and this technology provides a way to develop drugs that attack specific targets in cancer. Antibodies are a type of *targeted therapy*. Although they are "borrowed" from the immune system, most antibodies are not immunologic therapies *per se*, as they do not stimulate the immune system to destroy cancer cells. A number of such drugs now in use are specific for a variety of targets, such as the signals that tell cancer cells to grow and molecules that help a tumor develop its own blood supply. They generally must be delivered by the intravenous route.

This type of drug is, at present, limited by our knowledge of which targets should be attacked. As we learn more about cancer and are able to pinpoint good targets, this category of drugs is likely to grow and improve. One of their limitations is that they generally work best against targets that are outside of or on the surface of the cancer cell. They are not ideal for targets that hide deep inside the cells.

One variation on the antibody theme is to develop drugs that use an antibody as a *delivery vehicle* for the molecule that actually attacks a target within a cell. Such drugs attach a toxin or source of radioactivity to an antibody designed to destroy the cancer.

Small-Molecule Targeted Therapy

Better cancer therapy requires that we design drugs that specifically target the vulnerabilities of cancer but leave normal cells untouched.

Monoclonal antibodies are one way to do this because they attack only the invaders and leave other cells alone. However, antibodies have serious limitations. They are large molecules that generally cannot be made available in pill form, they cannot get deep inside a cancer cell, and they sometimes trigger allergic reactions. Increasingly sophisticated chemistry has enabled us to create entirely artificial chemicals that can also be quite specific in the targets they seek. They are called *small molecules* because they are much smaller than monoclonal antibodies and, as a consequence, they remain stable in the stomach and intestines. They can be made into pill form and can easily cross the outer and even the inner membranes in cancer cells to attack targets deep inside.

Small molecules have become the cornerstone of modern targeted cancer therapy. There have been a number of notable successes using small molecules. As we identify more and more good targets for such drugs, such as the particular proteins that drive cancer growth, we will see more drugs of this type developed and tested. Small molecules can be used against targets in any of the six hallmarks of cancer. For example, they can shut down the abnormal growth signal that drives the growth of many cancers. In many ways, small molecules are the chemical anticancer equivalent of antibiotics. Antibiotics are all small molecules, as are many other medications that treat heart disease, high blood pressure, and other common conditions.

Gene Therapy

Although gene therapy has gotten a lot of attention, so far it has not led to the production of successful cancer drugs. There are ongoing clinical trials of treatments in this category, so you may encounter gene therapy during your search for options. The goal of gene therapy is to replace a defective or missing gene, or to silence an overactive gene. This is an attractive approach because we know that genetic defects are at the root of nearly all cancers. However, inserting healthy genes has proven to be quite challenging. We can insert genes into cells quite successfully in the laboratory, but getting the healthy gene out of the lab and into cancer cells in a living human being is much more difficult. To fully succeed, we would probably need to insert the healthy gene into *all or nearly all of the cancer cells* in the human body, and even if only a small number of cancer cells evade this type of gene therapy, they can regrow and cause the cancer to recur.

Many studies are using specially designed viruses to deliver the healthy gene. However, even when the healthy gene is inserted into cancer cells, making sure that the new gene continues to be active and do its job has been another challenge. Sometimes, the cancer can turn off or silence new genes after they are delivered. Once this type of problem is worked out, we may be able to design custom drugs for each individual's cancer.

Gene silencing therapy is a mirror image of classic gene therapy. Some cancers are not missing a key healthy gene, but instead have the opposite problem: they are driven by defective genes. The defect leaves the gene in the *on* position continuously, and the overactive gene drives cancer growth, survival, or other critical functions. Drugs that are made of short sequences of genetic material (either DNA or RNA) can be designed to turn off such overactive genes.

We will come back to each of these categories in Chapter 9, when we discuss which current and emerging cancer drugs represent these broad drug categories.

Evolution of Medicine: From Systematic Knowledge to Evidence-Based Medicine and Toward Personalized Medicine

Finally, we would like to put all of these developments in a broader historical context. How do today's experimental approaches fit into the overall development of modern medicine? The modern era of American medicine began in the 1890s, with Sir William Osler, one of the four founding physicians of the Johns Hopkins University School of Medicine. Professor Osler created the first residency program for training doctors and was the first to insist that medical students be taken out of the classroom to learn hands-on at the patient's bedside. You'd think that would always have been the norm, but until then medical school focused only on theoretical learning; practical learning came later, after students had graduated. Osler systematically recorded the knowledge he gained through taking care of patients, as put forth in his landmark textbook, *The Principles and Practice of Medicine.*

Osler-trained physicians learned to systematically apply proven medical knowledge to the care of patients. This was a major step forward, but most doctors still largely relied on their own experience and observations. They did not yet trust evidence collected through experiments or clinical trials. It took a long time, but eventually this approach became the norm.

Today, the practice of medicine is largely built upon evidence of *clinical benefit*—the experience of real people who tried various treatments in clinical trials. The Scottish epidemiologist Archie Cochrane, through his book *Effectiveness and Efficiency: Random Reflections on Health Services*, published in 1972, is often credited with launching the *evidence-based medicine* movement. This wasn't very long ago. The term itself is even more recent—Dr. Gordon Guyatt coined it in the early 1990s. That's a lot of medical progress in about a century.

The practice of medicine is largely built upon evidence of clinical benefit*—the experience of real people who tried various treatments in clinical trials.*

Have we now reached the highest possible level of medical practice? Of course not. Today's evidence-based medicine has some major limitations, but it is likely to slowly evolve—or in some cases change rapidly—as biomedical knowledge continues to grow. Evidence-based medicine is good at defining what is best for large groups of people, but it cannot predict what treatment will work best for any one individual. Each person's uniqueness is reflected not only in our interests, personalities, physical abilities, appearance, and talents, but also in our health—including the way we experience cancer.

The average benefit seen in a clinical trial is not shared equally by all participants. Some are fortunate to be particularly responsive to an available treatment, others may get about the average amount of benefit, and still others may benefit less or not at all. Some may even be harmed by the treatment because they develop unpleasant side effects with little or no clinical benefit.

A Misconception You May Encounter

"Cures already exist, but they are being kept secret, so that doctors, hospitals, and drug companies can profit from the current standard treatments."

This one is one of those misconceptions that deserves the "You've gotta' be kidding" response. Our cancer drug market is huge, independent, and competitive. Large pharmaceutical companies compete with each other, and with thousands of small and medium-sized biotechnology companies. A new drug that is effective against cancer can generate billions of dollars in profit. The incentives to innovate are huge, and companies are highly motivated to develop breakthrough drugs.

On top of this, although it receives some funding from industry to operate trials, the academic research community is substantially independent. What motivates them? Most cancer researchers are passionately committed to curing cancer. Many have friends or family members affected by the disease. It is not uncommon for people to devote themselves to cancer research after a loved one experienced a battle with cancer.

Of course, they also want recognition as innovative and effective researchers. When they are successful, they can write journal articles and books! Further, these different groups (large, medium, and small drug companies, as well as academic researchers) exist all over the world. All of these competitors couldn't collude to slow progress even if they wanted to, and they don't want to anyway. All of the incentives are in the direction of innovation and accelerating—not slowing—advances.

A Misconception You May Encounter

"Most of the drugs used in trials in the United States are already approved in other countries."

Sometimes drugs are available outside of the United States first, but often they are not. The United States remains the world's leader in cancer research and, more often than not, Americans have the first chance to use new drugs.

As with treatment benefits, side effects are not equally distributed. Some patients tolerate treatment with few or no side effects, while others can have quite a difficult time. They may even choose to stop therapy because the side effects are too severe to tolerate.

Cancer research is moving toward being able to know in advance which treatments might be best for a given individual. Personalized medicine requires us to develop cancer treatments in parallel with specialized tests that are capable of predicting which patients are likely to benefit from specific treatments. Such drug–test couplets are becoming a reality. Two such treatments were approved for the treatment of cancer in 2011. You can read more about the development of personalized cancer treatment in Chapter 10.

There are many possibilities for identifying, managing, and curing cancer. Research is moving forward, and clinical trials are a key part of that research.

The Bottom Line

- Cancer uses the body's own nutrients to develop and grow.
- All cancers share several defining characteristics; these include:
  - Having its own growth engine; not depending on the body to send growth signals

  - The ability to ignore natural antigrowth instructions from the rest of the body
  - The ability to invade and spread throughout the body
  - "Immortality"—the ability to evade natural death
  - The ability to recruit cells of the vascular system to develop its own blood supply

- Major trends are defining areas for progress in the principal cancer treatments:
  - In cancer surgery:
    - More precise surgery
    - Less invasive operations
    - New technologies
    - Combining surgery with medical, radiation, and other cancer treatments
  - In radiation therapy:
    - More precise aiming of radiation
    - New types of radiation treatments
    - Combinations of radiation with other cancer treatments
  - In medical therapy:
    - Further development of chemotherapy with newer drugs and combinations of drugs
    - New ways to manipulate the hormones that drive certain cancers
    - More specific and targeted therapies through novel technologies, including, *artificial antibodies*, *synthetic small chemical molecules*, and *gene-directed therapies*
    - Harnessing the immune system to fight cancer
- All cancer therapy is likely to become more personalized (individualized) with treatments selected to match each person's unique cancer.

Part II

What Are Clinical Trials and How Are They Organized?

2

What Is a Clinical Trial?

A Brief History of Clinical Trials

The first documented clinical trial—undertaken long before this term had been invented—was conducted at sea with sailors suffering from what we now know was scurvy, a disease caused by a deficiency in vitamin C.

If you were at sea in the eighteenth century, you'd soon discover there was no medical center, no antibiotics, and no checkups on board, let alone health insurance or sick leave. When you signed up for a voyage, you literally took your life in your hands.

Perfectly healthy men became seriously ill or even died from scurvy during lengthy sea journeys. Nobody knew for sure what it was, what caused it, or how to cure it. The symptoms were horrific: bleeding ulcers, black spots on the skin, oozing mouth sores, teeth falling out, swollen limbs and joints, extreme pain, and loss of normal mental functions.

Many potential cures were tried, but with little or no benefit. As voyages became longer, scurvy became a bigger and more deadly problem. The success of some voyages depended more on the health and survival of crew members than on the navigational skills of the officers.

In the 1740s, James Lind, a Scottish doctor serving on an English vessel, came to suspect that scurvy was caused by a deficiency in the sailors' diet. Rotten, moldy, and worm- and insect-infested food was the norm. It's no wonder rum was so popular!

Dr. Lind's Plan

Lind proved what others had suspected: scurvy was caused by a nutritional deficiency that could be remedied with lemons and oranges. He had ample supplies of these hardy citrus fruits. To test his hypothesis (theory), he set up an experiment. He chose 12 men from the crew who were suffering from scurvy and divided them into six groups. Each group was given a different addition to their diet: with one including oranges and lemons.

Those eating the citrus fruit (the experimental group) were quickly cured. The sailors who did not eat the citrus fruit (the control groups) remained sick. This was scientific proof—by eighteenth-century standards—that scurvy could be prevented and cured with a simple dietary intervention. Lind's *clinical trial* was a success.

You would think that Dr. Lind would be widely hailed as a hero of the British Empire and glorious leader of medical science, but that was not to be his destiny. Few others were willing to give his *miracle cure* a try.

Scientific proof was no match for traditionally held opinions and biases. Captains, ship's doctors, and leaders of the British Navy ignored Lind's breakthrough work.

The story eventually had a happy ending, but it took more than 40 years! The British Navy and most other navies in the world finally adopted this simple dietary approach to preventing scurvy. Everyone now knows, of course, that scurvy is caused by a simple and easily preventable vitamin C deficiency.

Modern Medicine

We now live in an era of *evidence-based medicine.* Evidence of success, usually collected in clinical trials, is now expected before a treatment is adopted as safe and effective. We use such evidence to understand the risks and benefits of medical treatments and to make sound decisions about what treatments are best.

Clinical trials define the *gold standard* of care—the best treatment available. Medical science advances through clinical trials, even if progress is slow at times. Remember, it took more than 40 years for Dr. Lind's breakthrough results to become widely accepted. No area of medicine is more in need of advances than cancer care, and hundreds of novel treatments are currently being evaluated in cancer clinical trials.

Clinical trials define the gold standard *of care—the best treatment available.*

THE KEY INGREDIENTS OF A CLINICAL TRIAL

Although clinical trials have grown large, complex, expensive, and tightly regulated, the principles of a sound experiment are universal. The basic ingredients from Lind's eighteenth-century clinical trial remain the same in twenty-first-century clinical trials:

- *All trials begin with a hypothesis—an idea or a new theory—about what the researcher thinks will happen.* For example, Dr. Lind's hypothesis was that lemons and oranges might cure scurvy. The rest of the trial is all about testing the hypothesis. You prove it to be right, wrong, partially right, or partially wrong. Hypotheses can be as simple as this: the new drug ABC-123 will shrink cancer tumors (most new drugs begin with a boring name that resembles a license plate number!). Hypotheses can also be more complex: new drug ABC-123 will shrink tumors; it will also produce acceptable side effects up to a certain dose, above which the side effects will become unbearable, but it might work really well against some incurable cancers at a dose just shy of unbearable. You get the idea.

- *The trial is designed and carried out to test the hypothesis.* This is the *experiment*, the core of the trial (Dr. Lind used six groups of volunteers to test his hypothesis). The experiment, of course, has many parts, which we will explain in detail.
- *The results—what everyone is after.* Did it work? How well? A little? For which people? Can the results be duplicated with a larger group? Will it lead to a new approved medication or treatment, and, most importantly, did it or will it help *you*? At the outset, no one knows what the end results will be. That's why it's called a *trial.*

Even the most complex clinical trials are made up of simple parts and are fairly easy to understand, at least for those conducting them. Dr. Lind had a *hypothesis* that lemons and oranges would help sailors overcome scurvy. He gave lemons and oranges to some sailors and something else to others in order to find out if he was right (the *experiment*), and he learned that he was right (the *result*). *Hypothesis. Experiment. Results.* That's it "in a nutshell."

To understand what you are getting into if you're considering a clinical trial, you will need to understand the first two of these ingredients, *hypothesis* and *experiment.* Of course, you'll also want to know the third as soon as possible. It would certainly be nice to know what will happen before you even consider the trial. After all, why would you want to take a drug that may or may not work?

While you cannot know the results of a clinical trial that has not been completed, it's important to thoroughly understand *why* the trial is being conducted (the hypothesis) and *how* it's going to be conducted (the experiment). You'll also want to know how the clinical trial might benefit you: what is the expected—or hoped for—result. We will help you learn to ask the right questions of the right people to get these answers more quickly.

Clinical Trials Versus Standard Care

You may be thinking, "Why would I want to try a treatment that might or might not help me?" You may be right. *If there is an effective standard treatment that works for you, there is no reason for you to enter into a trial.* Here are some explanations that might help.

In many ways, clinical trials and standard care for cancer are similar. Both require you to visit doctors and nurses, take medications, have blood tests, have body and possibly brain scans, have regular physical exams, have needles inserted in tender places, and undergo many other procedures and indignities. For those of you who are just beginning cancer treatment, a great many unknowns will exist, in both experimental and standard treatments. After all, you have not done this before. You will encounter a lot of new information, face new treatments and unfamiliar tests, and have unexpected experiences. You could look at it as a new adventure in your life, although not an adventure you ever wished for!

Whoever came up with the term *standard* treatment didn't consider that, although it may be standard procedure for your doctor, nothing could be further from what *you* might consider standard. The whole process can be frightening.

Treatment for cancer—whether standard or experimental—usually involves side effects, expenses, testing, and a lot of your time. Standard treatments become standard when they are shown, in large clinical trials, to be better than the previously accepted standard. By *better* we mean that the entire group of patients who received the standard treatment generally fared better than the entire group of patients who received the treatment it replaced. This does *not* mean that every patient benefitted equally, and some people may not have benefitted at all. Standard treatments may involve a fair amount of uncertainty as to your personal outcome.

Even when you are beginning a treatment that is considered standard for your type of cancer, you will likely hear that a certain chance exists that you will benefit from it, often expressed as a percentage of people who remain cancer-free or whose cancers are under control a number of years after treatment. Hopefully, the chances of success are high, but they are almost never 100 percent, and often they are disappointingly low. When you participate in a clinical trial, generally less is known about the probabilities of various outcomes.

New treatments are needed because we don't yet have perfect cancer treatments. So, although there are more unknowns when you consider experimental therapy, they are often similar to those that you face when you receive standard therapy. It will be important for you to understand both options in order to make the right or best choice for you.

THE ELIGIBILITY CHECKLIST PROCESS

Despite the similarities, clinical trials are certainly not the same as regular cancer care. Trials are much more carefully regimented. Even before you get started, you will have to *qualify* to be in the trial. The doctor or study nurse has a long checklist of *eligibility criteria*. You may or may not be shown this list, but it's always part of any clinical trial.

This checklist—often 20 to 40 items long—lists all the criteria you will have to meet in order to qualify for a clinical trial. Thank goodness, we are not subjected to such checklists in most of what we do in everyday life! We'd never get anything done.

While the checklist may seem like the Great Wall of China standing between you and your hope of joining a study, it is there to protect you and to make sure that the study is carried out properly. Many of the criteria focus on ensuring that you are healthy enough or—in some cases—unhealthy enough to receive the proposed treatment. The criteria will likely include:

- Kidney function
- Liver function

- Heart function
- Blood counts

Other parts of the checklist are designed to make sure that all participants in the trial are similar enough, so that the experiment and results will be valid. It would be difficult to know how well a drug performed in advanced prostate cancer, for example, if the study participants had many different kinds of cancer in all stages. So, each trial defines the *patient population* for which it is designed. You will not know if you meet the trial's criteria until the qualification process—also called *screening*—is completed.

The rigid nature of a clinical trial does not end with your being admitted into the study. Once treatment starts, your care will follow a tightly scripted plan. The schedule of every blood test, scan, dose of medication, and doctor visit is dictated by the clinical trial *protocol*—it includes dates, times, places, and procedures. This can also be the case with standard cancer therapy, but although regular cancer therapy is thorough, it can be relatively flexible. Clinical trial therapy is closely controlled and monitored, because skipping a test or not taking a medication as prescribed could affect your care as well as the overall trial outcome.

The rigid nature of a clinical trial does not end with your being admitted into the study. Once treatment starts, your care will follow a tightly scripted plan.

Informed Consent

As discussed in detail in Chapter 7, clinical trials are tightly regulated and overseen by an independent oversight committee. One of the committee's responsibilities is to make sure that all participants are thoroughly informed about the trial they are considering. Participation in a trial will begin with the reading of a detailed, and often exhaustive, consent form.

You need to read the consent form and understand it—even if it seems long and boring. While the concept of *informed consent* is not unique to clinical trials, in routine care it often consists of nothing more than a conversation between a doctor and a patient. Not so for clinical trials. You get at least one conversation, sometimes two (doctor and nurse or study coordinator), and a volume of questions and statements in fine print. You not only have to read it, but also sign it. It's all quite a bit more formal than consenting to standard treatment.

Information About You

Finally, information about how you are doing with the trial medication goes into the medical record, as it does for standard care. It also goes into the study database, where it is combined with the experiences of all the other trial participants. This is referred to as the study *data*. Generally, you will have access to your personal results (although exceptions exist), but you probably will not be given information about results from the overall database. If you are given this information, it may be a long time before you receive it.

In addition to routine information, such as blood test results, the study may ask you to fill out surveys about how you are feeling, thinking, sleeping, eating, how your spouse is doing, and so on. Clinical trial studies often collect much more information about the daily routine in your life than doctors do in the course of routine standard care.

Whether there are five, 500, or 5,000 participants in the study, it is unlikely that you will know who else is in the trial. But you will know a lot about their type and stage of cancer, because it will be much like yours.

Statistics in Clinical Trials

Statistics are the tools used to interpret data from studies and discover if a real difference exists between two treatments. You need to have a basic understanding of statistics to evaluate what a clinical trial is seeking to accomplish. The same concepts will help you better evaluate standard treatments you may be considering. So, resist the urge to skip the following section and let us introduce you to a few key statistical concepts. This will help you know what to look for—and what to look out for—in order to understand your options and be aware of what you might expect from your treatments.

What Is Risk Reduction?

All treatments seek to reduce the risk of something bad—death, cancer coming back, or some terrible complication, for example. The way this reduction in risk is described can leave you more confused than informed. Ideally, your risk would be reduced to 0—meaning the treatment was a reliable cure. If that were the case, we would not need statistics very much. However, in almost all cases, modern cancer treatments work for some people and not for others, and risk reduction statistics are how we talk about the results. You may hear that drug "X" reduces the risk of cancer coming back by 40 percent. That sounds good, doesn't it? Not perfect, but it might make a big difference. Well—maybe, or maybe not.

In almost all cases, modern cancer treatments work for some people and not for others, and risk reduction statistics are how we talk about the results.

Most such statements focus on so-called *relative risk*. This is risk in the treated group compared to the control group (patients receiving some other treatment or no treatment). Whether, for example, a 40 percent risk reduction is great or not so great depends on the *absolute risk*—meaning the actual risk experienced by the control group. In many ways, an absolute risk reduction is probably the more accurate way to report results, but it never sounds as impressive.

As an example, let's say that women with a certain stage of breast cancer have a 90 percent chance of cure with surgery alone. In this situation, the *absolute* risk of cancer coming back is 10 percent. A *fantastic* drug comes along that reduces the risk of the cancer coming back by 40 percent! Sounds great, right? Maybe, but it may not be as impressive when you realize that the drug reduces risk from 10 percent to 6 percent. The risk was reduced by 40 percent, but it was small to begin with. When you start with a risk of 10 percent, a 40 percent reduction means that risk is reduced by 40 percent of 10 percent. This is equal to 4 percent.

This concept is subtle but it is really important. A 4 percent risk reduction in absolute terms could be quite significant, but it means that if we treat 100 women, 90 would have never suffered a recurrence in the first place, six would have had a recurrence anyway, and only four would have truly benefitted from the treatment—they would have had a recurrence without any treatment but won't because they were

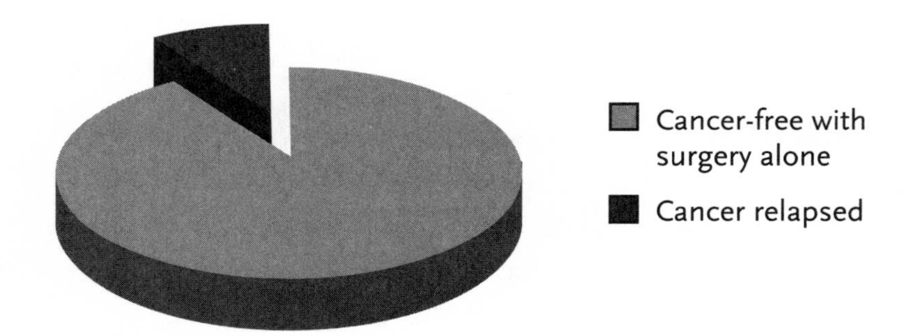

Risk of cancer relapse without additional treatment.

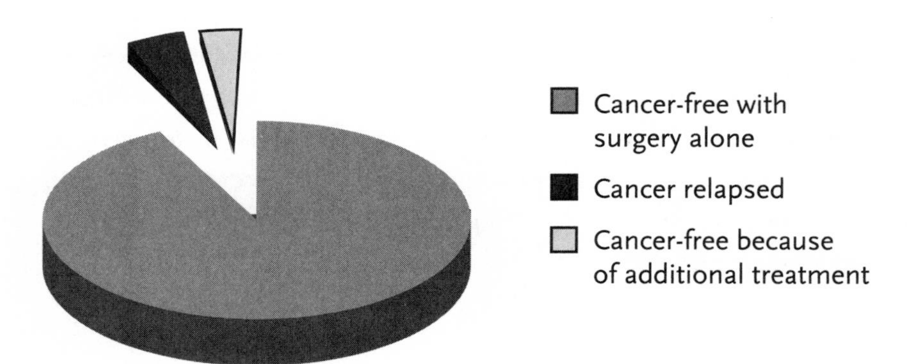

Risk of cancer relapse with additional treatment.

treated. It would be ideal, therefore, to just treat those four women and leave the other 96 alone! Someday, we may be able to do just that (see Chapter 10), but right now we can't tell in advance who they will be.

Understanding this can help you make decisions. A 4 percent reduction in the risk of cancer coming back may be a really important benefit for you. If so, the decision will be an easy one to make. However, if you have other health concerns, and the potential side effects of the new drug are severe, you might make a different decision. If all you hear is that the reduction is 40 percent, you might not even think about it.

When you see risk reduction numbers, ask yourself first: "What is the actual (absolute) risk to begin with?" Then ask: "Is the reduction an actual (absolute) reduction number, or is it a relative reduction in risk?"

What Is a Survival Benefit?

Many cancer treatments are not total cures, but they do improve symptoms and lengthen survival. The survival benefit may typically be reported in many different ways. You might hear that a treatment "improves survival by 30 percent." This might sound good at first, but the true value of this kind of a benefit can only be understood when you ask the question: "Thirty percent of *what*?" If you are dealing with a situation in which people with a certain type of cancer normally live several years, 30 percent better might mean surviving another year or more, and that could be good. On the other hand, some of the most lethal cancers are so aggressive that without treatment people may live only 3 to 4 months. A 30 percent improvement in this situation might mean less than a month. You can decide, of course, how worthwhile that might be, but only when you have a clear picture of all the factors involved and what you are actually trying to decide.

Sometimes, a survival benefit is expressed as months of survival. This is a little easier to understand, but it still can have some confusing wrinkles. This kind of survival number is usually calculated *at the median*, which is a single point in time when half of the patients remain alive. Because it focuses on a single point in time, it may not accurately reflect the overall survival advantage, which can be quite different for some patients than for others. Some people will benefit more than the average and others less.

Very few of us are absolutely average—in anything. Even a small average benefit could mean a large benefit for you as an individual, if you are fortunate. So, you may not wish to discard a treatment because of how it performs *on average*. You may wish to try it and see how it goes, and then drop it if it isn't benefiting you. Whatever you decide, always remember that you are almost certainly *not average*.

What Does "Significant" Mean?

When we hear the words *there was a significant treatment effect*, you would naturally assume that *significant* means large, important, or

A Misconception You May Encounter

"If I join one clinical trial, research rules would disqualify me from joining another trial."

Participating in one clinical trial does not disqualify you from future trials, as long as you meet the future study criteria. Many people participate in more than one clinical trial over time. Rules for trial participation do take into consideration therapy that you have received prior to joining a trial, and a prior treatment that you have received—either standard or experimental—might make you ineligible. If you already know you might be interested in a specific trial sometime in the future, look ahead and check to see if the treatment decisions you make today could get in the way later. For the most part, however, many other different clinical trials are available, and even if one particular study is off limits to you, another is likely to become a possibility.

A Misconception You May Encounter

"Researchers can get the same information about drugs through experiments on animals or computer simulations. Trials on people are not necessary."

We wish this were true. It is much easier and cheaper to do research with mice or on computers than it is to do it with human beings. A major effort under way, in fact, supported by the National Cancer Institute (NCI), to improve *preclinical models* of cancer. This basically means doing more studies using cancer-bearing mice that are good analogs of human cancer. Maybe one day we will get to the point where more research can be done in the laboratories and fewer human studies will be necessary. But, even if we do, there must always be a first human to try a drug. It is vital that this happens in a clinical trial, where the monitoring is extensive. It would be inconceivable and irresponsible to test a drug in animals and then make it generally available to people before careful human testing.

noteworthy. This may be true—but not necessarily. More often than not, *significant* refers to *statistically significant*, which means that the difference between the two groups of patients was statistically meaningful and unlikely to be random.

Statistical significance is an important concept. Without measuring the statistical significance of study results in cancer treatment, it is possible that any effects may not even be real but rather just chance. However, statistical significance is not enough. Another medical term—*clinically significant*—means "important to patient care." This is what we are after. If a small effect is statistically significant, it may still not be large enough for us to care much about it. Watch out for the word *significant*, and assume it's likely "statistics-speak" and not necessarily what you might think.

The Bottom Line

A clinical trial consists of these elements:

- The *Hypothesis.* Clinical trials begin with an idea.
- The *Experiment.* A clinical trial is an experiment designed to determine if the idea is a good one. You need to understand what the idea is and how the experiment is designed.
- The *Results.* What were the effects, good and/or bad? You will not know the results until after the clinical trial is over.

Clinical trials differ from standard care in several ways:

- Less is known about the effectiveness and side effects of experimental drugs than of standard drugs.
- Strict eligibility criteria determine who can take part.
- Formal informed consent and strict oversight is present.
- Predetermined schedules determine what happens and when.
- Information about how you are responding to the experimental agent and any side effects you experience will be combined with the experience of others and then analyzed.
- Statistics can be both accurate and misleading at the same time.
- Ask lots of questions about statistical results, so that you can understand just what all those numbers mean to you.
- Any statistic that is expressed as a percentage should prompt the question, *percent of what?*
- Ask your doctor how applicable any statistics are to your personal situation.
- ***Don't forget, you are not average. Almost nobody is.***

3

The Types of Clinical Trials: Four Phases and More

THERE ARE MANY KINDS OF CLINICAL TRIALS. Some are large; others are small. They may involve new medications, new uses for older medications, diet and lifestyle changes, surgery, and many other approaches. They may study prevention strategies, treatments for cancer, or interventions designed to improve quality of life. They may test a new treatment for the first time or make minor changes in an already approved treatment. However, despite the many variations among clinical trials, the way they are conducted *always* follows the same process. This is the organization of trials into *phases* based on how far along the drug or procedure being tested is in its development toward final approval as an effective therapy.

When your doctor tells you about a clinical trial, or you find one listed on the Internet, it is likely to be described as phase I, II, or III (and sometimes IV). What are these phases, and what do they have to do with you? The term *phase* refers to the steps in the drug development process. *Drug development* is the entire process necessary to create a drug, test it, and gain approval from the regulatory agencies. In the United States, this means that the Food and Drug Administration (FDA) must approve a drug before it can be offered (safely and legally) to doctors and their patients. The whole process can, and often does, take lots of money and lots of time.

Phase I: Safety Testing

In most cases, phase I studies might be appropriate for you if your cancer is not responsive to standard treatments. Since we don't know much about how successful the new drugs in phase I studies will turn out to be, proven treatments should be tried first. A phase I trial is a reasonable option to consider when proven treatments are not available.

Classic phase I studies are designed almost exclusively to test the safety of various doses of a brand new drug. The drug has already been analyzed, evaluated, tested on animals, and has shown promise in the laboratory for the treatment of cancer. Effectiveness may also be evaluated, but this is secondary to the primary goal of documenting side effects and safety. Phase I studies may be the first test of a new drug in humans. They use a dose that is *believed to be* safe—often 1/10 or 1/12 of the dose that is known to be safe in experimental animals—and determine whether this dose is safe in a small group of three to six patients.

Provided that no serious side effects occur, the dose is then increased and given to another small group of patients. This process, called *dose escalation*, is time-consuming and has to be carefully monitored. It continues until serious side effects begin to appear. When one patient experiences a side effect that is serious enough to stop treatment because the side effects are an important threat to the person's health and well-being, a small number of additional patients are often treated at the same dose to determine if this was a one-time event or whether a truly toxic or dangerous dose level has been reached. When more than one patient experiences significant side effects at a given dose, the study stops and the dose level one step below the toxic dose is declared the *maximum tolerated dose*, or MTD. A larger group of

When more than one patient experiences significant side effects at a given dose, the study stops and the dose level one step below the toxic dose is declared the maximum tolerated dose, *or MTD.*

patients may then be treated at this dose just to make sure. Once the MTD is determined, the main job of a phase I study is over.

Blood Level Studies

Phase I studies may also measure the drug levels reached in your system at each dose, whether taking the drug with or without food matters, and how quickly the body breaks down or *excretes* the drug (the time from taking the drug until it disappears from your system). This kind of testing is called *pharmacokinetics.* Despite what you might think, even most doctors don't love such tongue twisters, so pharmacokinetics is most often referred to simply as "PK."

The information collected in PK studies is important in understanding how the drug should be dosed and how it might be combined with other drugs—for example, whether it should it be taken three times a day, once a day, or once a week. It can take a lot of time and hard work for both you and the research team to figure this out. If you are a part of a study that is evaluating PK, you will be asked to have frequent blood draws after you take a dose of the drug. Often, a dozen or more blood draws are done over a 24-hour period. The blood draws are not evenly spaced, but rather are drawn close together at the beginning of the day and then spaced out more and more during the day.

Sometimes, you can spend the night at home and come back in the morning for the 24-hour draw, but sometimes you may be asked to spend the night in the hospital. In some cases, when a drug is processed slowly by your body, this may take more than 24 hours. The *good* news here is that usually a single intravenous catheter is attached to your arm or hand, and the blood is drawn over and over again from the same catheter. This means the number of needle pokes will be limited. You should bring a good book or two, and be prepared to be awakened one or more times in the middle of the night to give blood.

As you have probably figured out by now, phase I studies are not for everyone. While they provide the earliest opportunity to try the newest drugs, little is known about a drug when the first phase I study begins. It's not known whether the drug will prove to be safe in humans at any dose, whether it will be effective for *anyone*, and—even if it is effective—we won't yet know at which dose it works best.

Sometimes, a brand new drug proves quite effective and safe right away. Recent examples of this are the approved drug imatinib mesylate (Gleevec®) for chronic myelogenous leukemia, or the still experimental drug MDV3100 for prostate cancer. But for every success story, there are *many* phase I studies in which few or no patients experience improvements in their cancer status. Sometimes, the drug just doesn't prove effective at all. Occasionally, this can also happen with a drug that is later deemed to be useful. How is this possible? There are two main reasons:

- First, because safety is the primary concern, many patients may receive doses that are far too low to be effective before the effective dose can be determined. This can't be predicted ahead of time with certainty, but often turns out to be the case.
- The second common reason has to do with the patients and their cancers. Patients who participate in phase I clinical trials have often tried many different cancer treatments already. With each treatment that their cancer has managed to overcome, the cancer becomes more difficult to treat.

Variations of Phase I Testing

Not all phase I studies involve testing drugs in people for the first time. Sometimes, an established drug has to go through phase I testing again if the dosing amount or schedule is being significantly altered. For example, if a drug is normally given every 3 weeks, but researchers think that once a week dosing might work better, a phase I study to determine the right dose on a weekly schedule is necessary to make sure it's both *safe* and *effective*.

Sometimes, a phase I study can involve two or more well-established drugs.

Combining anticancer drugs is one strategy that is used to maximize the effectiveness of treatment. Drugs for cancer are often given at the highest doses possible, so a phase I study is necessary to determine safe dosage levels for each when two or more of them are combined for the first time. Although all phase I studies are conducted to ask a fundamental safety question, studies that examine established drugs in new dosing schemes or new combinations present fewer unknown risks than classic *first-in-human* phase I studies.

The Biologically Effective Dose

For some modern drugs, phase I studies are used to determine the dose at which the drug inhibits (or shuts down) cancer growth or other key features of cancer (see Chapter 1). As more drugs are designed to shut down specific cancer growth mechanisms, finding the *biologically effective dose* becomes more important than finding the highest dose possible. Doctors and patients hope that this will be a dose that does not cause severe side effects.

The good news for clinical trial participants is that there may be fewer side effects in studies of these drugs because they are more targeted. The *bad* news is that it's not always easy to determine if the expected biologic effect has occurred. In optimal situations, a simple blood test can be used, but in some cases, a repeat biopsy of the tumor is needed to measure the effect of the drug. Although biopsies may be necessary, they can be uncomfortable. Biopsies usually involve tissue samples extracted with a long hollow needle or a scalpel—a small sharp surgical knife. Sometimes, biopsies are done with *guidance.* This means that an imaging technique, such as ultrasound or a computed tomography (CT) scan, is used to give the doctor a visual guide to get the needle to the tumor. Almost always, a local anesthetic is used to numb the area and reduce pain. Sometimes, general sedation is also used to make the procedure more comfortable.

Why Would *You* Want to Participate in a Phase I Study?

Phase I primarily involves testing the safety of a new drug, so trials at this level are not likely to cure your cancer. A phase I trial could be a new and positive step, however, if your current treatment is not helping.

The positive features of participating in a phase I clinical trial include:

- You get the newest drugs or combination of drugs.
- You could get the first-in-human studies of a promising new drug.
- You could get new combinations of already proven drugs.
- You could get a proven drug being used for a different purpose.

There are some important negatives, including:

- There might be unknown side effects.
- The overall success rate is generally low.

Phase II: Initial Efficacy Testing: Does the New Drug Work?

Phase II studies are appropriate when no effective standard treatments are available. Some phase II studies may also be considered ahead of standard treatments, particularly if standard treatments are less than ideal (not always effective or associated with frequent side effects).

When people talk about participating in clinical trials, they are often referring to phase II studies. Once a phase I study has demonstrated that a drug is safe and well tolerated, and it has been determined which dose and schedule are appropriate for further testing, it's time for phase II testing. Phase II studies are the "workhorses" of cancer research. Their primary goal is to determine if a drug is safe and effective enough to challenge the status quo. If it is, then the drug will move on to phase III testing.

Types of Phase II Studies

Phase II studies are the "workhorses" of cancer research. Their primary goal is to determine if a drug is safe and effective enough to challenge the status quo.

You may encounter one of several types of phase II studies, including:

- Most commonly, all patients get the same drug or treatment, perhaps even the same dosage. Dozens or even hundreds of people with similar cancers are asked to participate in each phase II trial.
- Some phase II studies are *randomized*, as discussed in the next chapter. This means that you may be assigned randomly to one of the experimental treatments. These treatments might be two different doses of the same new drug, or possibly two or three new drugs that are all promising. The phase II trial will determine which drug will be used against the current standard drug (if there is one) in a phase III trial.
- In a trial where two or more different treatments are being compared to one another, each of these treatments is also referred to as an *arm* of the study. For example, if a higher dose and a lower dose of a drug are being tested, the study would be described as having two arms—a high-dose arm and a low-dose arm. One arm of a phase II study may include the current standard treatment, with no new drugs at all. This is done to provide a point of comparison for the new treatments.

What's in a Phase II Study for You?

If you're seriously looking for a clinical trial that might control your cancer or improve your condition, you may decide to participate in a phase II study. It might be a test of a new drug or a combination of existing proven drugs. In phase II studies, it is not yet known whether the medication or new combination is effective, or how effective it may be, but studies to date point toward the drug being beneficial in treating human cancer. If your current treatment is not helping you, this could be a good alternative. Participation in a phase II study could have one of several possible results:

- You could get better or even be cured—although a cure remains rare in many advanced cancers.
- Your cancer growth could be slowed and your quality of life improved.
- The results could be neutral—meaning there is no improvement and no harm has been done, but you receive close medical monitoring, and some of your treatment and testing may be free.
- As with any cancer treatment, you could be harmed if the treatment is not effective against your cancer or if you experience severe side effects.
- You will be helping to advance medical knowledge.

Phase III Trials: The New Treatment Compared to Standard Care

Phase III studies are appropriate if you are considering a standard treatment. They typically include the standard treatment and compare it to a new treatment that is thought to have a good chance of being better.

When things look good in phase II trials, indicating that the drug may actually be effective, it's time to take on the reigning champ—the standard therapy for your type of cancer—if there is one. Phase III studies are designed to determine whether the positive phase II results represent a true advance in cancer treatment. Typically, the new drug or new combination of drugs is compared to the current standard in a randomized study. Neither you nor your doctor gets to decide which treatment you get. That's up to the randomization process, which, as discussed in Chapter 4, is designed to ensure an unbiased comparison that will result in accurate and meaningful results.

Phase III trials allow for a direct comparison of the safety and effectiveness of a new treatment to the current standard treatment. For a new treatment to be approved by the FDA, it must have a real and substantial positive impact on patients' lives or their cancers. Therefore, phase III studies often measure how long people live, how long people live free of cancer, or whether a significant improvement occurs in quality of life. Mere changes in blood test values alone are not enough in a phase III trial. A successful phase III trial must meet the stringent standards of the FDA, which requires that new drugs be both *safe* and *effective* in order to be approved for general use.

Phase III trials allow for a direct comparison of the safety and effectiveness of a new treatment to the current standard treatment. For a new treatment to be approved by the FDA, it must have a real and substantial positive impact on patients' lives or their cancers.

At first, it might seem that smaller studies should be able to tell us whether a new drug is safe and effective, so we can skip the huge effort, cost, and time that phase III studies require. Phase III studies often involve hundreds or thousands of patients. However, the history of cancer treatment is full of promising results from small studies that did not survive the true test of a randomized comparison to the current standard. Finding effective medications is a complicated, time-consuming, and difficult undertaking.

Why Would *You* Volunteer for a Phase III Clinical Trial?

Large numbers of patients are involved in phase III studies, and a good chance for positive outcomes exists because the new medication has shown strong indications of effectiveness, and the standard therapy is already known to be effective. In a Phase III study, the current best medication on the market—if there is one—is tested against the new medication. These comparisons are always large and randomized. This should be a win-win for everyone. Your risk of harm is relatively low, and your chance of a positive outcome is quite good. Your treatment is always closely monitored, and some elements of your treatment may be provided free of charge.

Phase IV Studies

Similar to phase III studies, phase IV studies are appropriate if you are considering a standard treatment.

Phase IV studies are a lot like phase III studies, but their objective is to further refine the use of an *already approved drug*, not the initial testing of a completely new drug for which approval is being sought. Phase IV studies may be designed to learn more about the safety of a new drug, such as long-term side effects that may not have been determined in a phase III trial. A new dose or treatment schedule of a drug may be undergoing testing against the previously approved approach. Phase IV studies may also be designed to confirm the benefits seen in prior studies. Such studies are often required by the FDA when the initial approval of a drug was based on an *accelerated approval* process. Therefore, phase IV studies are quite similar to phase III studies. There are many examples of drugs that were studied in phase IV trials after they were approved.

What's in a Phase IV Study for *You*?

Phase IV studies are conducted with approved drugs, and relatively modest improvements are expected. This level of trial involves the least risk of any type of trial, but it is also less likely to include the latest innovative drugs. They tend to be win-win studies. You'll get a proven treatment or medication. The main question is whether you will get a good treatment or an even better one. Phase IV studies, however, are not an automatic gateway to the newest drugs.

Phase 0 (Zero) Studies

The phase 0 study is relatively new. It was designed to speed up the relatively slow process of testing a new drug by beginning with a small short-term study whose purpose is to test whether or not a drug does what it should do—biologically—when given to a human being, and whether it is worthy of further evaluation in a phase I study. For example, if a drug is designed to shut down a particular cancer protein, it wouldn't stand a chance of helping patients if it were unable to shut down the intended target. Phase 0 studies are typically charged with making sure that the drug is able to get to where it needs to go in the human body and shut down its target. If it does this, larger studies involving more patients who are given the drug for a longer period of time can go forward to determine if the approach is successful in shrinking or eliminating cancer.

Typically, a group of five to ten participants take an experimental medication for a period of a week or two. Extensive testing and evaluation during this period help determine whether the medication is promising and should be studied further in a phase I study. Tumor biopsies may be used to check whether the drugs are doing what they are designed to do in the cancerous tissues. Although phase 0 studies typically involve the latest drugs, they are not necessarily designed to effectively treat your cancer. Consider all of your options carefully, and be sure you understand whether or not there is a possibility a particular phase 0 study might be helpful.

A Word About Other Types of Studies

Most of the clinical trials you hear about involve some type of experimental medication or treatment—something that may slow, manage, or cure your cancer. But other trials don't involve anticancer medications or treatments. Although the focus of this book is primarily on studies of new cancer treatments, you may also encounter studies of supportive care

Most of the clinical trials you hear about involve some type of experimental medication or treatment—something that may slow, manage, or cure your cancer. But other trials don't involve anticancer medications or treatments.

treatments, such as new antinausea or anemia treatments, exercise, or other treatments directed at improving symptom management or quality of life. Other studies may be devoted to improving long-term survivorship after cancer treatment. Such studies focus on reducing or eliminating the long-term effects of having had cancer and being treated for the disease. These studies do not directly target your cancer, but they may examine important treatments that have the potential to lessen the burdens of living with cancer. Similarly, new diagnostic procedures, such as new scanning methods to detect cancer or new blood tests to monitor it, may also undergo evaluation in clinical trials. The general approach to these studies is quite similar to trials of new cancer drugs.

Why Would You Consider Participating in a Clinical Trial That Doesn't Involve a Treatment Intended to Directly Treat Cancer?

Achieving a better quality of life while living with cancer is important. For example, trials in this category have enabled us to markedly reduce some of the dreaded side effects of chemotherapy, such as nausea. Some interventions that improve quality of life while living with cancer can also extend life. For example, trials involving strength training resulted in an increased lifespan in cancer survivors, including those with incurable cancer.

The Bottom Line: The Advantages and Disadvantages of Various Types of Clinical Trials

How can you decide on a type or phase of clinical trial in which to participate? The following table summarizes the advantages and disadvantages of the different phases of clinical trials.

The Advantages and Disadvantages of Various Types of Clinical Trials

Advantages	Disadvantages
Phase I Studies	
• You will have access to the newest drugs being developed around the world. • Everyone gets the new drug, but not necessarily in the same dose. • The drugs are provided free of charge, and some other costs of treatment may be free.	• Often, little is known about the drug before testing starts. • The dose you receive may be too high or too low to be safe or effective. You may never know if it might work for you in a different dosage. • The drug may prove ineffective or have unpleasant or even serious side effects.
Phase II Studies	
• You will have access to the nearly newest drugs that have already undergone some human testing. • The optimal dose or an optimal dose range is already known from the phase I study. • Everyone gets treated and, most of the time, everyone gets the new drug.	• Limited information about the safety of the drug is known, because only a small number of patients have taken it. • The efficacy of the drug is not known—will it actually slow, reverse, or cure your cancer? • The standard treatment could be better, so you will want to know all your options before volunteering.
Phase III and IV Studies	
• Only promising drugs make it to phase III, because the FDA is awaiting proof, so that the drug can be approved. • The drug is still relatively new, but it has already been tested in many people.	• There may only be a one in two chance that you will get the new treatment. If you don't, you would get the same treatment that has been the standard until now. This is not necessarily a disadvantage, but something that you need to know ahead of time. • You have to be comfortable with letting a computer decide which treatment you get—you won't get to choose.

4

Randomized Trials and Placebos

NOBODY WANTS TO FEEL *RANDOMIZED*. We want to make choices and control our own destiny. Read on to learn more about randomization and why, in some cases, it might be the right choice in your particular situation.

Participants in clinical studies are often randomly assigned to various groups in the study and will receive slightly or completely different treatments. It could be that different strengths of the experimental drug are being tested, or that two or more different drugs are being tested and compared. Being randomly assigned means that you don't have the choice of which group you're assigned to. Your doctor doesn't have a choice either, and neither of you may know what drug or what strength of the drug you are receiving until the study is over—if ever. Phase I and many phase II studies generally do not involve randomization, but nearly all phase III and IV studies and some phase II studies do.

Randomization: Letting the Computer Decide

Let's say you're walking in the forest, come to a fork in the path, and aren't sure which way to go. You flip a coin. Heads, you go right; tails, you go left. This is an example of randomization—unless it's a two-headed coin, of course—or you can use the Yogi Berra method: "When you come to a fork in the road, take it!"

When participants are randomly assigned to the various treatment groups in a clinical trial, it is done by using computerized randomization, random number programs, or tables of random numbers. This helps to ensure that the ultimate results, whatever they may be, will be scientifically sound.

There is evidence of using random assignment more than 2,000 years ago, but the modern medical use of randomization dates to the middle 1800s. Random assignment to treatment or nontreatment groups helps make the results of studies more accurate and informative. It allows us to know that a new treatment is not just good, but is definitely better than one we used before. It can tell us that a new treatment is less effective than the standard treatment, equivalent to it, or that it has significant side effects that limit its use. More than 50,000 documented studies have used randomization as a part of the research protocol.

Randomization in Today's Clinical Trials

Will being randomly assigned be of benefit to you? Maybe yes; maybe no. This can't be known ahead of time, because a randomized trial cannot exist without *equipoise*, which means that *no one* knows which of the treatments being randomly assigned is better. If the best treatment were already known, there would be no need for randomization, or even for the study. *Equipoise is a core ethical principle of clinical trials.*

What if an effective treatment already exists? How can there be randomized trials in that situation? As you probably know by now, few medical treatments are perfect; most treatments can be improved upon. They can be made even more effective, or perhaps they can be made safer with fewer side effects. If an effective treatment already exists, a randomized trial will often compare the current best treatment to a modified treatment (one that has a high probability of not being worse and has some chance of being better). This might mean comparing a standard drug to a standard drug plus a new drug. It might mean examining a shorter course of chemotherapy or a less invasive surgery than the current standard to see if the same benefits could be achieved with less damage.

Almost all of the cancer treatments available today have gone through such a comparison. You might be surprised to know that *subtraction* (meaning shorter duration of a less toxic therapy) has been almost as common as *addition* (more drugs may be better) in advancing care. For example, thanks to studies that compare less to more treatment, we now know that most men with testicular cancer can be cured with only 12 weeks of therapy, rather than the 6 months or longer that used to be standard. We also now know that many women with breast cancer only need a *lumpectomy*, in which only the tumor is removed and the rest of the breast can be left intact. As a result, the number of total mastectomies has been dramatically reduced. More about these advances and randomized trials that have changed cancer therapy can be found in the next chapter.

Comparing Active Treatment to No Treatment

Sometimes, no standard treatment is available. The standard treatment is therefore simply to wait and watch. This is often the case when we are trying to *prevent* cancer from occurring. There are not many proven cancer prevention strategies—with the exception that quitting smoking is probably the single best and most effective cancer prevention strategy there is!

People with cancer may not have standard treatment available to them. This can be terrible news; for example, when a cancer is aggressive and nothing is known to be effective. But it isn't *always* bad news. Sometimes, the standard treatment is observation when a cancer is slow-growing and either the available treatment is worse than the disease itself or currently available treatments could be used later with the same benefit. Observation has few side effects, so it can be a good strategy when a cancer is not an urgent threat. For example, low-grade, low-risk prostate cancer is often watched to determine whether it is aggressive enough to be treated. Many men can live their full lifespan with untreated low-grade prostate cancer. In situations in which the standard treatment is observation, a randomized trial might compare a new treatment to no treatment, or to a placebo combined with the *best supportive care.* It can be difficult to get used to the idea that a trial comparing a new treatment to no treatment is medically correct and ethical, but in some situations that's exactly the case.

Our society is inherently action-oriented, and we tend to err on the side of doing *something.* A common reaction is that doing something must be better than doing nothing. This is not always so. There are many examples of studies, particularly in the prevention area, in which taking a supplement or a medication did not reduce cancer risk—and may have caused some side effects. *Doing* is not always better than *watching.* Ethical oversight of trials ensures that if one of the options in a randomized trial is *doing nothing* or some variation on the theme, then there truly is equipoise and we really don't know that doing *anything* is helpful.

Blinding and Placebos

Some randomized trials are *blinded* while others are not. Blinding can be accomplished by using a *placebo*—a biologically neutral substance packaged to look like a real drug. Although often referred to as a *sugar pill,* many placebos are not pills. They are simply inactive compounds packaged to look, feel, and appear like the active drug or the other therapy being studied in a clinical trial. They may be an injection, intravenous infusion, capsule, a cream, an inhaler, a skin patch, or any other form used in the active treatment.

Blinding is not always a matter of giving one group a drug and the other group an identical-looking sugar pill. For example, actual acupuncture treatment can be compared to sham (fake) acupuncture.

As another example, two different surgeries can be compared to one another, with a particular element of the surgery changed, although the wound looks the same to both the patient and the evaluating physician.

Most blinded studies are *double-blinded*, meaning that neither the patient nor the doctor knows which treatment is being used. However, sometimes double-blinding is not possible, and a study is *single-blinded*, meaning that only the patient doesn't know which treatment she is receiving. This would be unusual in a drug study, but if two surgical techniques are being compared to one another, the surgeon certainly needs to know! Sometimes, blinding is impossible. If a study were comparing surgery to radiation, for example, some really crazy and elaborate steps would have to be taken to blind the study, including sham surgery and sham radiation!

Being in a blinded study can be frustrating. We all want to know what we are getting. We shy away from mystery meals because it is human nature to want to know and understand what we are taking into our bodies. We may not always make good choices with this knowledge—we smoke, eat unhealthy foods, and drive too fast—but at least we know what we are doing when we make these choices. We are in control, or at least we think we are. Not knowing what medication you are taking can also be uncomfortable for the physicians participating in the trial. They would prefer to know which treatment you are getting. It's their job to take care of any side effects and inform their patients about what is happening, and not knowing which drug you are taking makes this more challenging. "I have no idea what I just prescribed to you" is not a phrase a doctor would be likely to utter comfortably in most situations, and it isn't likely to make a patient feel confident either!

Randomization and blinding are hard to carry out. They increase the complexity and cost of running the trial and make everyone involved a little uneasy. So, why do we do it? Because, like randomization, blinding helps ensure that the results are valid and credible. The central idea behind randomized studies is that they allow us to eliminate most or all of the other variables that might explain the ultimate outcome of the study. As a group, the people who receive one of the treatments in the study should be similar to those who receive the other treatment; they should have a similar state of health, similar diets, and take similar medications.

Everyone who participates in a clinical trial is unique. By assigning all of these unique folks to two study groups through randomization, we hope the differences will average out and the two groups will end up being fairly similar. Then, if the study yields a positive result—for example, survival is longer in one group than the other—we can feel confident that the new treatment is the reason for the improvement.

Another important benefit of a blinded study, made possible by a placebo, is an accurate accounting of the side effects of a new drug. You probably already know that side effect listings on medications are far from an exact science. *Adverse medical events* (side effects) can happen to anyone, but they are more likely to happen to those of us who are older and fighting cancer. The doctors on the front lines who are trying a new drug often don't know if the nausea, pain, fatigue, rash, and other side effects are from the new drug or from something else—including possibly one of the many drugs the patient is already taking, a virus, stress, bad luck, or other factors.

Using a placebo can give us information about which side effects occur more often with the new drug than with the placebo.

Benefits Can Be Hard to See Without Blinding

The benefits of randomization can be lost to a great extent when a study is not blinded and patients in one group begin to behave differently from those in the other group, possibly because they know what treatment they are getting. There are many ways this could happen. Patients might quit the study early if they did not get the assignment they were hoping for. They could start making healthier choices, take different medications, and see their doctors more or less frequently because they know what treatment they are receiving.

Doctors might treat their patients differently if they knew what group they were in. For example, they could be less thorough in looking for side effects in the group receiving the standard treatment or a placebo. All of these choices, whether conscious or not, could undermine the integrity of the study and produce misleading results. Blinding helps preserve the scientific integrity of studies and makes sure that the treatments we use are truly beneficial.

Blinding is important in most randomized studies because even measures as black and white as overall survival can be influenced by the choices patients and doctors make. It is particularly important in studies that focus on the relief of symptoms and quality of life.

The Appropriate Role of Placebos in Clinical Trials

Many people with cancer are understandably concerned that they might get a placebo instead of a real treatment. This is often the first question the physician or researcher hears when a clinical trial is brought up as an option, "Will I get the real thing or just a sugar pill?"

The fundamental principle that defines when placebos are appropriate is rather simple: *if a treatment that works is available, a placebo cannot be used instead.* Period—end of story. Research *is not* and *cannot* be about withholding effective treatments from patients with cancer. A placebo can be used in two research situations:

- A placebo is often used when *no effective treatment is available*, and the standard treatment would be observation or perhaps supportive treatments designed to lessen symptoms but not treat the disease. This is often the situation in prevention studies. This may also apply to people with advanced cancers, when all of the active standard treatments have been exhausted, or in cancers for which no effective treatment has yet been identified.

- A placebo can also be used when *an effective treatment exists and this treatment is being given to all of the patients in the study*. In this type of study, the placebo is *added* to the known effective treatment to allow a comparison between the standard treatment *and* a combination of the standard treatment plus a new drug of unknown effectiveness.

The Placebo Effect

The placebo can be considered one of the oldest of medicines. Despite their inert nature, placebos have been associated with important improvements in the health and well-being of the people who have used them.

The degree to which placebos work varies considerably, depending on what disease is being studied, but it stands to reason that if we are going to devise a new drug, it should produce more useful results than a mere look-alike. According to the American Cancer Society, placebos have an effect on about *one in three* patients. Often, the result is a reported improvement in a symptom or in quality of life. Sometimes, it can actually be a new side effect. How placebos work is not fully understood, but they may represent, to some extent, the importance of the mind–body connection.

Many cultures have relied on strengthening the mind–body connection to promote healing. The placebo may be one way this happens in Western culture. A placebo can reinforce patients' belief that they will get better, and so they actually do. In general, placebo effects are seen as symptoms or something else that people feel.

How placebos work is not fully understood, but they may represent, to some extent, the importance of the mind–body connection.

In some studies, the positive effects of the *placebo group* are greater than those of the *experimental group*. These studies show the amazing (and mysterious) power of placebos, and that without them we may have drawn a different conclusion and promoted an ineffective treatment.

Placebos in History

Placebos have been around for thousands of years and have a rather illustrious history. Placebo is Latin for *I will please.* Does a placebo *please you* or make you feel better? It seems that it often does.

Throughout most of recorded history, there were few effective, proven medications of any kind. Historically, almost all medical treatments were medications with no known healing quality. They might as well be called "placebos." Nobody knew for sure whether the recommended treatment had any medical effect, and in many cases, it probably did not. But the patient might have improved anyway.

Healers, elders, and medical practitioners have long known that sometimes people get better, or at least feel better, when they use substances or other treatments that clearly have no medicinal powers, as far as we know. By the eighteenth and nineteenth centuries, doctors were able to treat some illnesses more or less successfully (recall the story of Dr. Lind and the dreaded scurvy from Chapter 2).

Beginning in the nineteenth century, doctors and scientists began to test existing medications by comparing them to placebos. By the late twentieth century and continuing into the twenty-first, clinical trials comparing multiple treatments—sometimes using a placebo in one arm of the study—have been common, carefully regulated, and often successful.

The most important fact for you, as a cancer patient, is to know that the use of placebos in clinical trials is tightly regulated by ethical standards and overseen by multiple regulatory bodies. If any effective treatment is available, you won't get a placebo alone, and if a placebo is to be used in the study, you'll certainly know ahead of time that this is a possibility.

Chapter 7 provides more detailed information about how research studies are regulated and how participants are protected.

Why Are Randomized Trials So Large?

Randomized trials often involve hundreds or even thousands of patients. The largest ones may involve tens of thousands. Why do they need to be so large? Wouldn't it be faster to get answers if fewer patients were required to carry out a clinical trial? It certainly would be, but having too few patients involved may also mean missing the answer or inadvertently declaring a good treatment ineffective because its benefit could not be detected as a result of the small number of people involved. The size of a trial is determined by complex statistical calculations. The differences between treatments are often small, and they only become *statistically significant* with larger numbers of participants.

The most important determinant of how many people need to participate in a clinical trial is the size of the expected benefit of a new treatment. Simply put, if the old treatment didn't work at all, and the new treatment cured everyone (we can only wish), it wouldn't take very many patients to discover that the new treatment is a tremendous advancement. After the first 20 or 30 patients it would be obvious to everyone—and statistically valid, as well. At the other end of the spectrum, if the expected improvement is a 20 percent extension of life, but not a cure, a large number of participants may be needed to prove it. Such an improvement could make a tremendous difference to a lot of people, so it's important to find it. But, from the perspective of statisticians, such a difference is relatively small, and random chance could get in the way if too few patients participated in the study. The bottom line is that studies are no larger than absolutely necessary to detect the expected benefit.

What Happens If a Study Shows a Benefit Even Before It Is Finished?

As you now know, equipoise must exist before a randomized trial starts. We must genuinely not know which treatment is better. Hopefully, we will get the answer to the basic question asked in the study when the trial is completed.

That's the way it is most of the time, but what happens if the answer becomes obvious even before the trial is complete? Is anyone paying attention to that? Yes!

Every large randomized trial must have a *data safety monitoring board* (or *committee*), often referred to as the DSMB or the DSMC. This is a small group of scientists and statisticians—often three to five people—who are independent from the study, are sworn to secrecy, and have total access to the data as the study proceeds. Their role is more fully described in Chapter 7, but in brief, the job of the DSMB is to stop the trial early if there is clear evidence that one of the treatments is better than the other. Very few study participants even know that such a board exists and that its sole purpose is to protect them.

Did I Get the Best Treatment?

Although randomization makes for good science and good medicine, with results that can be trusted, it still leaves one open question for individual participants. "Did I get the best possible treatment option?" The answer is that we don't actually know. In order to participate in a randomized trial, you have to accept and believe that if we did know, randomization wouldn't be an option. If you are not equally comfortable with all of the options in the various arms of a randomized study, then a randomized study is not for you. If a well-established, effective treatment is available, and it is not a part of the randomized trial you are considering, you may feel more comfortable receiving the standard treatment first and considering studies later, if needed. If you *do* participate in a randomized trial, you won't know in advance if you received the best possible treatment, but that is not to say that you will never find out.

The hope in carrying out randomized studies is, of course, that one of the arms will prove better than the other. That's progress. When the study is done and the results are published, you will see the results and know if you got the most effective treatment. It's just not possible to know the outcome in advance.

HOW CAN I BE SURE I GET THE *NEW* TREATMENT?

There are several ways that may allow you to have access to a new treatment being tested. The first does not involve the completion of the study. Some randomized studies allow a *crossover*. In this type of situation, participants receiving a randomized treatment later receive the treatment that was given to the other group of people in the study. This is of particular interest to patients who missed out on the new drug and were randomly assigned to the standard treatment. You will be told before you start whether the study design will allow a crossover.

Sometimes, there is no possibility for crossover. For example, crossover is generally impossible in situations in which no measures are strong enough to be accepted as proof that a drug is beneficial, except for length of life (survival). Crossover also does not guarantee access to a better treatment. At the time patients switch treatments, it will not yet be known if the newer treatment is, in fact, better.

Some randomized studies allow a crossover, *in which participants receiving a randomized treatment later receive the treatment that was given to the other group of patients in the study.*

Once it is clear that the new treatment is better, there are three ways to get the new drug as soon as possible. First, if a DSMB stops the trial early because the results are good, the researchers conducting the trial have a moral obligation to give the new treatment to all the study participants who did not receive it in the first place, if possible. When an announcement of an early study closure due to the success of a trial is made, it is often accompanied by a plan to provide the new drug to all study participants who did not receive it in the study.

You might be offered an option with a title such as *compassionate use protocol* or *early access program.* When a new drug is clearly a winner, and the company who owns it is going to the FDA to seek approval, it can sometimes offer the drug on a limited basis to patients who are likely to benefit. Be sure to ask about this type of opportunity.

Finally, a drug that is clearly beneficial will eventually be approved, at which time it can be prescribed to anyone. Although the approval process has a reputation of taking a long, long time, the reality is that the approval process can be rapid if a randomized trial has demonstrated a compelling advantage. The FDA generally has 6 months to respond to an application, but it has approved new drugs in 3 or 4

A Misconception You May Encounter

"I don't want to be randomized. If I could only get the new drug, I will be much better off."

Randomized studies are done because there is hope that the new drugs will be better. Otherwise, there would be no point to a study. It is natural for you to hope that the new drug will be a winner. The truth is, however, that randomized studies are also done because we really don't know which drug is better. There are many examples in which we learned that the standard treatment was better than the new drug being tested.

If you are randomly assigned to the standard treatment, you can take comfort in knowing that you are receiving the best treatment currently available, and that you are probably being monitored more closely and carefully than if you were being treated outside of a study. Your experience, along with the experiences of the other participants, will not just be recorded on your personal medical record. It will also become a part of a study that hopefully advances care for all cancer patients, including, possibly, you. You may also be able to get the new drug a little later, especially if it's a clear winner, or have an opportunity to participate in another trial that gives you access to another new, experimental drug.

months when the benefit is clear-cut. If there is an obvious winner with a real benefit, everybody involved will work as fast as possible to make it available to all patients who need it.

The Bottom Line

- Randomized trials usually compare a new treatment to the current standard; if there is no currently available treatment, it will be compared to a placebo.
- Randomization is only permissible when we do not know which treatment is better.
- Randomization ensures that patients in each treatment group are similar, so that when a difference is seen at the end of the study, we can be highly confident that it's because of the new treatment and not because of differences in the participants.
- Blinding makes sure that patients who are assigned to different treatments by randomization don't make different decisions about the rest of their health care and skew the results.
- A placebo is an inactive substance that is made to look like the active drug. It's not always the classic *sugar pill.* It's made to match (look like, and sometimes taste and smell like) the active drug being tested. Thus, it might be a patch, an intravenous solution, or take many other forms.
- Placebos allow patients and their doctors to remain *blinded* to the study treatment. This reduces the risk that the results might be biased by choices made by the patient and physician as a result of knowing what treatment the patient is receiving.
- When a study has a placebo-only arm, it means that the standard approach would be no treatment, which is essentially the same as a placebo.
- When an effective treatment is available, a placebo can be added to it to test a new combination of treatments; however, in such cases, all patients still get the proven treatment.

- Placebos can have their own positive and negative effects. They are not well understood, but may represent the mind–body connection and the effects of believing that you are getting a valid treatment that will help you.
- All randomized trials have a fully independent monitoring board. If it becomes obvious that one treatment is better or worse than another, the board has both the right and the obligation to stop the study early and make these results known.
- If you participate in a randomized trial, you will not be able to choose your treatment. You must be willing to accept randomized assignment to determine which group you will be in.
- When you choose to participate in a randomized trial, there are several ways to get the new treatment if it proves more effective than a placebo or standard treatment:
  - The study may allow a *crossover*. This means that if your cancer begins to progress, you might get a chance to try the other treatment. It does not mean that the other treatment is necessarily better, but you may get a chance to try both the old and the new if there is a crossover. Be sure to ask whether the study you are considering includes a crossover.
  - If a study is a resounding success and it's stopped early, the patients who received the standard treatment often have immediate access to the more effective new treatment.
  - If a study is successful and the company plans to apply for drug approval, sometimes an expanded access protocol allows people who did not receive the active treatment in the trial—or even people who were not a part of the trial—to get early access to the new treatment. This is often available at the research centers that participated in the trial.
  - A strong winner usually gets approved quickly after completion of a randomized trial. Watch for the new drug to become available.

5

Clinical Trials That Have Changed Cancer Care

SOME CLINICAL TRIALS CHANGE THE WORLD, even as others fail to make much of an impact and fade away. In this chapter, we're going to share our selection of ten clinical trials that advanced the field of cancer treatment and made a stunning difference in the lives of many patients. Some of these top ten studies established revolutionary new treatments, some eliminated unnecessary treatments without sacrificing effectiveness, and some debunked long-held beliefs. This progress would not have happened without the vision of the researchers and the courage of the patients who volunteered to become study participants.

Some studies establish revolutionary new treatments, some eliminate unnecessary treatments without sacrificing effectiveness, and some debunk long-held beliefs.

Top ten may seem a bit pretentious, since these selections are based solely on our judgment. We didn't conduct a survey or take a vote among our peers. Of course, there are hundreds or even thousands of other studies that have resulted in positive life changes for people with cancer. Read about the extraordinary trials we selected and decide for yourself.

Surgery Cures More Women with Breast Cancer When Supported by Chemotherapy

Early Treatment Saves Lives: Three-Drug Chemotherapy Cocktail (CMF) Versus No Treatment

We now take it for granted that adding effective medications to surgery and radiation can save the lives of women whose breast cancer has spread to their lymph nodes. But this was not always the case. Although *local* therapies—surgery and radiation—can be quite effective, without additional treatment, microscopic amounts of cancer may be left behind. When these *seeds* grow, they can become a life-threatening relapse of the original cancer. Effective cancer medications do not eliminate this risk, but they can decrease it substantially.

Chemotherapy has changed and become more effective, over time. CMF—a three-drug chemotherapy cocktail containing cyclophosphamide, methotrexate, and 5-fluorouracil—was the standard treatment for years, but now we can do better. The drug combination approach, which is now called *adjuvant therapy*, has endured and become a cornerstone of modern breast cancer care. When Gianni Bonadonna started the first such clinical trial in 1973, the idea that women should be randomly assigned to chemotherapy or observation after they completed their surgery and radiation was revolutionary. In fact, as treatments have improved, they have been shown to benefit not only women whose cancer has already begun to spread by invading nearby lymph nodes, but also those whose risk of recurrence is not as high. Today, only women who have a low risk of *relapse* and a high probability of cure with surgery (sometimes followed by radiation) are treated *without* some form of adjuvant therapy. Countless women who would have succumbed to breast cancer are still alive because of the innovative thinking of researchers and the courage of the women who volunteered for this and many subsequent studies.

When Less May Be More

Less Surgery Can Be Better: Lumpectomy Versus Mastectomy in Breast Cancer

It's a good bet that everyone with cancer would prefer less rather than more surgery if they could be confident that there would be no compromise in the quality of care. Not all studies challenge the status quo by adding a new drug. Instead, some ask the question, "Are we doing too much?" Breast cancer surgery, which at one time was extremely extensive, has evolved to become less and less invasive as the result of clinical trials that asked this question.

William Halstead performed the first *radical mastectomy* in 1882. This extensive breast cancer surgery included the removal of chest muscles and lymph nodes in the neck, leaving women significantly disfigured. Since the early 1970s, modern surgeons have systematically scaled back the extent of mastectomies to the minimum necessary to do the job. Part of this progress was aided by the development of effective chemotherapies and radiation, which supported surgery and allowed surgeons to be less aggressive, thereby causing less disfigurement.

A number of studies have contributed to this effort, but one landmark study challenged conventional thinking more than any other by comparing a *full mastectomy*—removal of the whole breast—to a *lumpectomy*—removal of only the tumor (lump)—followed by radiation. Halstead would have been truly surprised. Removal of muscles and neck tissue was long gone by the time this study was done because it had been shown to be unnecessary. This trial further demonstrated that—for many women—removal of the tumor alone and leaving most of the breast untouched can be both safe and effective. Women now have a much better chance of surviving breast cancer *and* keeping their bodies intact in the process.

Does Surgery Really Help Men with Prostate Cancer?

To Treat or Not to Treat: Surgery Versus Observation in Prostate Cancer

If it's difficult to make a decision about the clinical trial you might be considering, imagine a trial that allows randomization to decide between treating your cancer with aggressive surgery and leaving it in your body entirely untreated. This sounds more than a bit crazy doesn't it? Most trials ask you to consider two different drugs or two different surgical treatments, but major surgery versus no treatment at all is extraordinary.

There has been a lot of debate about whether men with localized prostate cancer benefit from aggressive treatment, or whether they should be left untreated. The theory was that the cancers dangerous enough to require treatment are already too far along to be removed successfully, while those that could be treated easily were destined to grow so slowly that they never needed treatment in the first place—a real "catch-22" dilemma. This theory did not survive clinical trials showing that the treatment of localized prostate cancer with surgery cut the rate of progression, cancer spreading, and death by nearly 50 percent. Studies established the effectiveness of active treatment for many localized prostate cancers. Thus, many men are now spared the life-threatening consequences of advanced prostate cancer through effective early treatment.

A Sum That Is Truly Better Than Its Parts: Combining Chemotherapy Drugs

A Chemotherapy Cure Is Born

With today's growing focus on biologic agents that carefully target a cancer's biologic weak points, it's easy to forget that standard chemotherapy remains the mainstay of treatment for many cancers and that it has saved countless lives.

Standard chemotherapy remains the mainstay of treatment for many cancers and has saved countless lives.

Early in the history of chemotherapy, physician-scientists discovered that treating cancers with one drug at a time could produce some improvements, but that these successes were often short-lived. Cancers treated this way develop resistance to the drugs used against them. To overcome this problem, scientists hypothesized that attacking the cancer from several directions at once might work better. Clinical trials proved this theory correct by testing combinations of chemotherapy drugs given together.

The first four-drug chemotherapy cocktail was called MOPP, named for the four drugs involved: nitrogen mustard, vincristine, procarbazine, and prednisone. This combination was used to treat Hodgkin's lymphoma, a cancer of the lymph nodes, and it converted the disease from deadly to often readily curable. The regimens currently used have been refined to cause fewer side effects, but the underlying principle is the same. Hodgkin's lymphoma can easily withstand one chemotherapeutic drug at a time, but four drugs together prove overwhelming to the cancer in a large majority of patients. Similarly, a combination of three drugs: cisplatin, etoposide, and bleomycin, changed the face of testicular (or testes) cancer treatment. Today, more than 90 percent of patients diagnosed with this cancer are cured. The three-drug regimen first published by Dr. Einhorn in 1984 is still the gold standard.

Location, Location, Location

Sparing Your Organs Is Always a Noble Goal

Just as in real estate, a key feature of cancer is its location. Some locations render the cancer easily detected and readily treatable, while others mean that treatment might be difficult or lead to significant disability.

Cancers of the larynx are an example of tumors in a difficult location. They are often detected early because patients note hoarseness in their voice, which can result from even small lumps on the vocal cords. Removing the larynx is effective, but it leaves the patient unable to speak. Fortunately, carefully conducted studies have shown that a combination of chemotherapy and radiation can cure the cancer as effectively as removing the larynx. People can now be cured of this type of cancer *and* keep their voice!

Similar approaches have allowed limbs to be spared for patients with sarcomas. Anal cancer can be treated in this manner to avoid the need for a *colostomy* (a bag attached to the abdomen that collects stool). There are many other examples in which carefully planned clinical trials have allowed a curable cancer to remain curable and kept the patient physically intact during the process.

A Successful Revolution: Targeting Mutations That Cause Cancer

Taking Away Cancer's Accelerator

For decades now, a central tenet of the "war on cancer" has been that we must understand what went wrong to cause a normal cell to become cancerous. We believe this understanding will allow us to create drugs and other treatments that will attack cancer precisely and effectively, while sparing the patient most side effects.

Imatinib mesylate (Gleevec®) is just such a drug. It targets a genetic mutation that causes a type of leukemia called *chronic myelogenous leukemia* (CML). This mutation, called *BCR-ABL*, acts like an accelerator that is stuck in the "on" position, driving the growth of leukemic cells with nothing to stop it. Imatinib binds to BCR-ABL and turns off the "go" signal. At the time it was developed, few physicians and researchers had confidence that targeting a cancer mutation would actually work. The prevailing belief was that we should focus our scientific efforts on chemotherapy.

Dr. Brian Druker believed otherwise. In his phase I clinical study of imatinib, 53 of 54 patients demonstrated dramatic improvements. Through a series of clinical trials, imatinib has revolutionized the care of CML and several other cancers that involve similar defects. This remarkable advance allows people with CML to live their lives with few, if any, of the side effects of chemotherapy. In the world of cancer research, it proved that treatments targeting specific defects responsible for cancer cell growth can produce remarkable results. Today, much of cancer research focuses on this approach (see Chapters 1 and 10).

Hormones and Cancer Prevention

Cancer Prevention That Actually Works!

It makes good sense that research should focus more on preventing cancer in the first place than on treating it after it occurs. If you read the popular press, it might seem that little is being done to prevent cancer, but this is not true. There have been, and continue to be, considerable efforts in cancer prevention.

Unfortunately, cancer prevention trials are difficult, large, and expensive to carry out. They take a long time because cancers don't develop on a regular schedule. They require a large number of volunteers because many people—thankfully—will *not* develop cancer during the study. Interventions to prevent cancer must be quite safe and cause few side effects in order for healthy individuals with no symptoms to adopt them. No one would accept chemotherapy, for example, to prevent a cancer that does not exist and may never come. Finally, we still know

It makes good sense that research should focus more on preventing cancer in the first place than on treating it after it occurs.

too little about how cancer starts and develops to create effective prevention strategies.

Despite these challenges, two large trials, the Breast Cancer Prevention Trial (BCPT) and the Prostate Cancer Prevention Trial (PCPT), showed that hormonal treatments can reduce the risk of developing breast and prostate cancer. In the case of breast cancer, the estrogen blocker tamoxifen was compared to a placebo in women at increased risk of breast cancer. In the prostate study, finasteride, a pill that reduces the conversion of testosterone to its more active form, dihydrotestosterone, was compared to a placebo in men over the age of 55. Age is the most important risk factor for prostate cancer and—similar to the women who participated in the BCPT study—these men were also at an elevated risk of prostate cancer. These studies showed that both men and women with a high risk of cancer have the option of doing something that may postpone or even prevent the problem from occurring.

Boost Your Immune System

Activating the Immune System to Enhance Its Ability to Combat Cancer

Physicians and researchers have long suspected that the human immune system has the power to combat cancer, and a number of studies have provided encouraging clues as to how this may occur. This approach has had some successes, but they have been few and far between. In studies of *immunotherapy*—a treatment that works by stimulating the immune system—only a small percentage of patients have benefitted, but some of them have benefitted greatly. Unfortunately, we have no good way of knowing which immune activators will work for specific individuals. This makes immunotherapy difficult to use routinely.

A recent study of ipilimumab (Yervoy®), a monoclonal antibody that strongly activates the immune system, reported a near doubling of survival of patients suffering from melanoma, the most deadly form of skin cancer. Ipilimumab was quickly approved and made available to extend the lives of men and women who suffer from this aggressive cancer. Results such as this point the way forward and reaffirm our confidence that targeting the immune system is a promising strategy to fight cancer. Perhaps one day we will be able to harness the immune system to prevent many types of cancer.

Debunking a Medical Bias

More Is Not Always Better

There are still many biases and unproven beliefs in cancer treatment. They can become particularly harmful when they involve toxic and complex therapies that have not been adequately tested. This was the case with using bone marrow transplants to treat the side effects of the high doses of chemotherapy used to treat breast cancer.

Success with chemotherapy to reduce the risk of breast cancer recurrence led to the hope that more chemotherapy could yield even better outcomes. A frequent limitation to how much chemotherapy can be given is damage to the bone marrow, where blood and immune cells are made. Too much chemotherapy can irreparably harm the bone marrow, causing severely low blood counts. A bone marrow transplant can help get around this limitation. This surgical procedure involves removing a sample of the patient's bone marrow, delivering the chemotherapy, and then replacing the bone marrow. A small, nonrandomized study in patients with breast cancer suggested that high doses of chemotherapy—when combined with a bone marrow transplant—could yield excellent results. Patients and doctors flocked to the new treatments, and properly randomized studies were not conducted before a large number of patients had been treated with this approach.

By the time the randomized study results were finally announced, breast cancer had become one of the most common cancers to be treated with a bone marrow transplant. The results of the new studies "blew a big hole" in the conventional wisdom. Several randomized trials all told the same story: bone marrow transplant *did not* improve outcomes. More is not always better.

Bone marrow transplants are almost never a part of current breast cancer care. We now know that, although chemotherapy can be quite helpful, a ceiling exists beyond which more is not better, and can actually make a situation worse. The focus of research has changed to newer treatments that more specifically target the genetic defects that cause breast cancer. These new treatments are being added to the most effective chemotherapy regimens.

When Our Basic Beliefs Are Challenged

Surprising and Unexpected Results
May Challenge Popular Beliefs

For many years, beta carotene—a form of vitamin A—was thought to have important anticancer properties. The available data supported this belief, which was so widely held that not one but two huge randomized studies, the Alpha Tocopherol and Beta Carotene (ATBC) trial and the beta carotene and retinol (CARET) trial examined the potential of beta carotene to reduce the risk of lung cancer in smokers. Just about everyone believed this would be a "slam dunk."

Nobody expected the results. Not only did beta carotene fail to reduce lung cancer, but those who took it were at significantly *greater risk* of developing lung cancer than those who didn't. It would be hard to believe the results if they had not been proved in large-scale double-blind trials that involved tens of thousands of participants.

We now know not to recommend beta carotene as a supplement to smokers—and maybe not to anyone else. We are reminded once again that, until proper studies are done, we won't know everything, and that a lot of what we *think* we know might just be completely wrong.

The Next Breakthrough Study—What Will it Be?

Will it be the one you're about to begin? You never know. Some trials fail to achieve their goals, some advance the field a little, and some usher in revolutionary change. It's not possible to know any of this in advance. As illustrated by the breakthrough studies described above, sometimes the hoped-for innovation really happens, and sometimes the result is entirely unexpected. Researchers, physicians, and patients would do well to keep their minds open. We have much to learn, and we know that progress and cures sometimes come from unlikely directions.

Some trials fail to achieve their goals, some advance the field a little, and some usher in revolutionary change. It's not possible to know any of this in advance.

The Bottom Line

Successful clinical trials are the source of new knowledge about what works and what does not work in cancer treatment. There is no single formula for success. But we do know that the most important and successful trials have:

- Led to the development of new drugs and drug combinations for advanced cancers
- Advanced and improved surgical techniques

- Provided methods to prevent or delay the development of cancer
- Harnessed the immune system
- Often challenged conventional thinking

Not all studies change the way cancer is treated, but we can never know the potential benefits until the trials are conducted, the work is evaluated, and the results are known.

Part III

Deciding Whether to Participate in a Clinical Trial

6

Is There a Clinical Trial That's Right for Me?

Deciding Whether to Participate in a Clinical Trial

Deciding whether to make a clinical trial part of your care, or whether to continue standard treatments, is not straightforward. We can't tell you what to do, but we will suggest an approach to thinking this through. Some circumstances that could lead you to consider experimental therapy include:

- No effective standard therapy is available, but ongoing research and experimental treatments are available.
- Standard treatments do not have to be completely ineffective for people to consider a clinical trial. In some cases, standard therapy is not very effective and/or it causes severe side effects, and you're thinking of trying something different, even if it is experimental.
- Standard therapy is reasonably good, but there is room for improvement and you're always looking for something new and better.
- There are no other alternatives; you've already tried all the standard therapies.

What Should You Know Before Choosing a Clinical Trial?

Here are some of the question you should ask your doctor and research team:

- What are the possible benefits for me?
    - Short term
    - Long term
- What are the possible risks for me?
- What reasonable options do I have other than a clinical trial?
- Do the possible benefits outweigh the possible risks?
- What will happen to me during the trial?
- Will it involve any painful treatments or procedures?
- How long will it last?
- Will I still be able to take my other medications and continue the treatments I'm currently receiving?
- Who will be in charge of the trial?
- Who will pay for it?
- Who can I talk to during the study when I have questions or concerns?
- Will I have to alter my lifestyle?

What Potential Benefits and Risks Should You Consider Before Choosing a Clinical Trial?

Clinical trials can provide several benefits:

- You will receive closely supervised care.
- Leading specialists in the field will develop your care plan.
- You may have access to new drugs before they become available to the broader patient population.
- Your health will be closely monitored.

- You will play an active role in your own health care.
- You could be among the first to benefit from a new drug.
- You will be making a contribution to medical science.

Clinical trials may also have risks:

- There may be unknown side effects—even long after the trial is over. This is not likely, but it is possible.
- The treatment may be ineffective, and you will receive no benefit.
- The treatment may work for some, but not for you.

The Effects of Attitudes, Emotions, and Reality in Choosing a Clinical Trial

Although we focus much of our discussion on the *facts* that you need to know, your decision-making process will also involve your *feelings* and *emotions.* Beyond the medical reality of a cancer diagnosis, just knowing you have cancer is likely to have a significant emotional impact on you, your family, and your friends. The process of coming to accept your diagnosis, maintaining your life as normally as possible, and then thinking about clinical trials can be emotionally difficult.

Beyond the medical reality of a cancer diagnosis, just knowing you have cancer is likely to have a significant emotional impact on you, your family, and your friends.

Once a person receives a diagnosis of cancer, it is common to go through a period of *denial*—"There must be a mistake; this can't be happening to me." This is often followed by despair—"What's the use; there's no hope."

You may feel so discouraged after your diagnosis that you can't really focus on anything else, at least for a while. It's normal to initially feel depressed and anxious, "I've got incurable cancer, and I'm going to die!" It's a horrible feeling, regardless of whether it's true or not.

If it turns out your cancer is *not* curable, you and those around you could feel absolutely devastated, at least at first. It might seem like the end of the world as you knew it. Your feelings are real to you. They may not be logical, rational, or reflect reality—that's why they're called *feelings* and not facts—but they have a major impact on what you think, how you act, and what you decide to do or not do. This includes whether or not you choose to join a clinical trial.

Actually, there might be real survival benefits in how you mentally and emotionally cope with cancer. Calling yourself a *survivor*, for example, has a certain determined, optimistic sound to it, and this is a good place to start.

According to the National Cancer Institute (NCI), about half of all people with incurable cancer also have to cope with serious emotional distress and anxiety. People with cancer can experience *post-traumatic stress disorder* (PTSD), just as accident victims or soldiers in combat can. Cancer survivors commonly experience fatigue, especially if they have recently undergone surgery, chemotherapy, or radiation therapy. Fatigue can make it more difficult to make decisions and take actions that might benefit you.

"I Just Want to Be Left Alone!"

Whatever you are feeling, it is normal for you and is probably shared by many others with cancer. You're not the only one who has a lot of strong and confusing feelings. It's common to want to be alone and avoid the sympathy and concern of others. You may even avoid your family and closest friends. Isolation might help but, more likely, being alone will increase your stress. These feelings may persist for a few weeks, a few months, or even longer. You may feel sad, happy, angry, and discouraged—all at the same time. This emotional roller coaster can keep you from getting the help and support you need, and from making important decisions. Try not to let this happen. Tell yourself you're in control and then *take charge*! This might not be easy, but it is good advice and worth a try.

The American Cancer Society (ACS) suggests some things you can do to help manage worry and stress:

- Talking about your feelings can help relieve worry and stress.
- Relaxing with deep breathing and other techniques can be helpful. Doing it regularly works best.
- Allowing yourself to feel sad and frustrated without feeling guilty about it is perfectly okay, and you have every right to feel this way.
- Choosing the right person to talk with is important. This person might be a good friend, family member, or a spiritual counselor.
- Spiritual help is useful for many people.
- If the worry persists or gets worse, get help from a mental health professional.

Cancer Support Groups

People with cancer who participate in support groups report a better quality of life than those who do not. There are support groups in many areas where you will find others who are facing the same problems and can provide helpful support. Discussing your concerns about joining a clinical trial with your support group can help you get a more realistic idea of just what to expect. You just might learn something that will be helpful.

How do you find out about support groups? First, talk with your doctor and share your feelings and fears. Your doctor and medical team can offer support, suggestions, and perhaps a lot more help than you ever imagined. Most likely, they can put you in touch with a support group or someone who can help you find one. Unless you tell them, no one will know how you feel, what your fears are, and what you need.

Many hospitals and cancer treatment centers sponsor support groups. There are also numerous online groups and most of them are legitimate, but don't give out too much of your personal information until you're sure. If a group asks for money to join, be cautious. Look on the major cancer websites, such as the American Cancer Society (ACS) site, www.cancer.org or the Association of Cancer Online Resources (ACOR) site, www.acor.org, for support group suggestions.

CHOOSING THE *RIGHT* TRIAL FOR YOUR NEEDS

Everyone involved in a clinical trial has a vested interest in the outcome of the trial:

- The *pharmaceutical companies* are in business to test, prove the efficacy of, and market new treatments. Their mission and business success depends on the successful development of new drugs. *They* want the medication to work.
- The *hospitals and doctors* want the drugs to be effective so they can help patients. They are responsible for conducting trials of new drugs under strict controls to safeguard patients, and to determine whether new drugs and treatments are both effective and safe. *They* want the medication to work.
- *You* are interested in managing or curing your cancer. You want a treatment or drug without nasty side effects that is going to manage your cancer, lengthen your life, and improve your quality of life. *You* want the medication to work.

Look for a trial that meets your needs, as well as meeting the needs and expectations of the pharmaceutical companies and medical community.

I'm Interested. What Do I Do Next?

Maybe you're thinking, "I've read about dozens of trials, and they all sound okay, but how will I know if one is *right* or at least *better than the others* for me? Who will help me find trials, get information, and get treated? How long is too long to wait—I don't have forever, you know! Where do I start? What if my cancer is rapidly getting worse? How do I know if I would even qualify?"

More than 6,500 cancer clinical trials are available at any one time. For more common cancers, hundreds of studies may be under way. This is good news, of course. When there are multiple studies, there will be many new ideas on how we might improve treatment and find cures. But, for you, it can make getting usable information a formidable challenge. Fortunately, by using the strategies we describe, you will not need to evaluate each and every trial.

Start Close to Home

A conversation with your own doctor is always the best place to start. Tell your oncologist that you are interested in experimental therapies or clinical trials. You may find that your physician or hospital is offering one or more clinical trials, or she may be aware of nearby programs that are involved in clinical trials for people with your needs and interests.

Even if you end up doing most of the research on your own, your doctor will be a key source of support and information. At a minimum, she will need to share information about you and your cancer with those conducting the clinical trial. You will certainly want the support of your doctor and medical team.

Know Your Disease State, Stage, and Prior and Current Treatments

Before you begin searching, you need to know several key pieces of information about your cancer and the treatments you've had so far. The more you know, the more quickly you'll be able to narrow your search to what you want and not waste valuable time.

Every clinical trial is carefully designed for specific groups of patients. For example, phase I studies of brand new drugs are typically looking for patients with advanced cancer that has spread (metastasized) and is not responsive to standard treatments. We don't know much about how successful these new drugs might turn out to be, so proven standard treatments should be tried first. If nothing else is available and you don't have a proven standard treatment to fall back on, a phase I trial is a reasonable direction to go.

Many trials focus on treatments for advanced cancers, but trials for patients with earlier-stage cancer are also available. For example, trials of *adjuvant* treatment test cancer treatments that are administered shortly after the primary surgery or radiation, in the hope of reducing the risk of disease recurrence. Some patients may be cancer-free after initial treatment, but have a type of cancer that suggests a high risk of relapse. They may be interested in and eligible for this type of study. Patients who are candidates for standard therapy—at any point in the course of the disease—may want to try clinical trials examining new approaches that researchers hope will improve on standard treatment outcomes.

Clinical trials are available for patients at all stages of cancer, and for those who have had a broad range of prior treatments. However, the studies for one stage or situation will probably not be the same as those for another. Knowing your stage and treatment history is absolutely necessary before you can sift through all the possible trials to identify those of relevance and interest to you.

Searching Online—The Basics

The single most complete resource for clinical trials in cancer is offered through the NCI at www.cancer.gov. This website provides comprehensive, up-to-date, and reliable information about a range of cancer topics, including standard treatments, research programs, and clinical trials.

Pick the *Clinical Trials* tab on the www.cancer.gov website, then choose the *Find a Clinical Trial* bullet. This opens the *Search* screen. The specific headings may change a bit from time to time, but with a little patience you'll find your way.

Start your search by giving some basic information about yourself and your cancer. Some of this information is needed to begin, and more will be required as you read about the trials you are considering. Prepare for your search in advance by assembling the following information:

- Your location, including your zip code; how far are you willing to travel for care?
- General health information; for example: Can you take care of yourself? Can you drive? Do you have diabetes or heart disease in addition to cancer?
- Your type of cancer; often you can pick from a list.
- Subtype of cancer; this may or may not be relevant for your cancer, but some cancers have distinct subgroups that make a difference in how they are treated. For example, in breast cancer, the presence or absence of hormone receptors determines whether hormonal therapies might be used successfully. Different studies are designed for cancers that have or do not have such receptors.
- Stage of your cancer; this may not be required, at first, but can really help narrow down your search.
- Prior treatment history; this may not be needed for your initial search, but it's important as you start reading about trials. Prior treatment history, combined with cancer stage and your general health, will determine whether you are potentially eligible to participate in a specific trial.

You will also want to collect information about the trials that are currently available. There may be hundreds if your cancer is common (there are many trials for breast cancer, for example) or just a few (for rare types of cancer, such as biliary tract cancer). Some of the items you will want to jot down as you are reviewing trials include:

- Who is conducting the trial? Are they well known and reliable? Ask your doctor.
- Is the trial currently active and accepting new participants?
- How do I find out if I am eligible, or how I can become eligible?
- What experimental treatments will be used?
- Will my insurance cover basic costs (see Chapter 8)? Remember that, in the U.S., Medicare always pays for medical care in approved

trials, the same way that it pays for routine care. Coverage may vary with other insurers, and differences can exist from state to state.

- How long will the trial last? Most, but not all trials have a specific time frame.
- How do I apply?

Advanced Searches

The NCI search engine lets you keep things simple. For example, you can enter just the type of cancer you have and see what is available. It also lets you get much more detailed. If you have a rare cancer, a basic search may be the place to begin. But, for more common cancers, you will quickly discover that dozens and perhaps hundreds of studies are available nationwide, although many may not be relevant to your specific situation. It's time to narrow the search and find the studies that may be appropriate for you.

Here are the steps you can take to narrow your search. Remember that the NCI's search engine is always being modified, so it may look a little different than this, but the principles will be the same.

1. Select the *type of cancer* that you have. Cancer is always named by where it started in your body. For example, if you have breast cancer that has spread to the liver and bones, it is still breast cancer—not liver or bone cancer.
2. Once you have entered the type of cancer, a box will open up with choices about the *subtype and stage.* This is different for every cancer. Look at this carefully and read the whole list. You may fit into more than one category. If you are not sure, ask your doctor which of the categories best describes your current situation.
3. Next, you have the opportunity to think about *where* you would like to look. You may want to start with your zip code and indicate how far you are willing to drive. You can also leave this part of the search blank. If you leave this blank, you will see what trials are available all over the country. There are also other useful options

for limiting the location of trials you want to consider; for example, you can restrict your search to your city, your state, or even a particular hospital or institution where you feel comfortable.

4. Selecting the type of trial can really help you get focused. Take a look at all the options. The first is *treatment.* If you have cancer and are looking for cancer treatments, check this box. This will eliminate a lot of studies that may be looking at prevention, detection, new diagnostic tests, cancer risk, and other things that may not be right for you. Of course, if you are interested in prevention studies, or you are looking for studies that focus on symptoms but not on treating cancer directly, you can select these boxes instead.
5. You will have the opportunity to *select a specific drug.* Most people should leave this search field blank. You probably don't want to limit yourself to one or two drugs at first, but instead you should look at everything that is potentially available. This option is also useful if you have heard of a particular drug and want to see what studies are under way with it. You will be able to pick from a list, so you won't have to double-check the spelling of a recently invented cancer drug—which is helpful, as they are often tongue twisters.
6. The next field lets you narrow your search by *treatment type.* This can be a bit confusing because you just had the chance to select the *type of trial* (see No. 4 above). While the type of trial is fairly general (for example, treatment or prevention), the treatment type is quite specific. It can let you focus on fairly general treatment types—such as chemotherapy or surgery—or be specific with a subtype of surgery, radiation, or medication class. Many people leave this search field blank, at least at first. However, if you know for sure that you are looking for trials that involve radiation, surgery, or laser procedures, this can be a good way to eliminate all the other trials you are not interested in.
7. The *key word or phrase* field lets you try searching using words that describe what you are looking for. The results can be quite variable depending on what words you choose. General words, such as

"chemotherapy," will not help the search very much. For most people, it's probably a good idea to leave this field blank when you start your search.

8. The *trial status* is set to show all active trials. You can narrow your search to phase I, II, III, or IV trials, if you already know you are interested in a specific phase. Most importantly, you can also check the *new trials* box. This will show you only trials added in the last 30 days. This feature can be enormously helpful if you want to track any new developments after your initial search. Checking this box allows you to avoid repeating the entire search process and just see what is new. If you log in once every 30 days to check for new studies, you can stay fully informed about what has become available.
9. Finally, if you are interested in a trial at a *specific location* run by a specific researcher, or sponsored by a specific agency or organization, the NCI site allows you to narrow your search accordingly in the trial ID/sponsor box.

If you need help with online searching, your spouse, children, or grandchildren might be a source of assistance. You can also seek out a friend who may have gone through the process, or ask a librarian or aide at a senior center. The possibilities are endless—you just have to ask!

Many other websites provide information about clinical trials. You can search online for clinical trials provided by private organizations, specific hospitals, or even those available in other countries. Be aware that some sites may require you to enroll or even pay a fee to participate. Think carefully about those options.

I've Done My Homework . . . Now What?

Hopefully, your search has yielded some good and conveniently accessible options, not too many and not too few. Print or save the descriptions of the trials in which you might be interested and read through them. You should be able to get a sense of whether you are likely to qualify and what is involved. The descriptions do not include every bit of information about a study, but they do provide quite a bit of detail. You can expect an overall description of the study, a listing of its goals and objectives, and the ever-important *eligibility criteria* that are used to determine which patients will be invited to participate.

Despite having narrowed and refined your search, you will probably find some trials that don't meet your objectives and others that may sound interesting, but for which you don't qualify. Once you've done this initial homework, it's time to make an appointment with your oncologist, bring in your findings, and get an honest opinion about how the various studies might fit your circumstances. This could also be a good time to get a second opinion.

You can contact a study center at any time. The study details (which can be found at www.cancer.gov/clinicaltrials) nearly always include the name of a knowledgeable contact person with an e-mail address and a phone number. Don't hesitate to take advantage of the chance to gather more information. The investigators want to hear from potential volunteers, because they often need more. If you think you have found a good fit, but have a few questions before you make a trip to the study center, give them a call. At some point in the conversation, the questions will go from general questions about the study to the specifics of your individual needs and situation. It is likely that they will want to see you in person for an evaluation, to make sure the study is appropriate for you and vice versa. However, you can save yourself quite a bit of time and hassle by getting some basic questions answered before you make an appointment.

With experimental therapy, you may never be 100 percent sure about the choices and decisions you make. But the more homework you do, the more confident you'll be. If your inner voice still says, "Something's just not right here," ask more questions.

The Bottom Line

- You may wish to consider a clinical trial if:
  - No standard therapy is available.
  - Standard therapy is not very effective or causes severe side effects.
  - Standard therapy is reasonably good, but there is room for improvement.
  - Standard therapy is no longer working, and there are no other alternatives.
- Give yourself permission to experience all of your feelings when you are facing the diagnosis of cancer. Get help when you are ready. If considering a clinical trial is too much right now, perhaps you will want to consider it later.
- Finding a trial that fits your needs, is close by, is available, and has room for you can be a time-consuming and complex undertaking, but it is made much easier by the NCI's website, www.cancer.gov/clinicaltrials.
- The more detailed you can be about what you are looking for, the more likely it is that your search will yield a manageable number of study options.
- Knowing your cancer stage, prior treatments, and general health will help you take your first steps toward determining whether you might qualify for a clinical trial.
- Don't hesitate to get help. Talk to your doctor, get a second opinion if necessary, and call or e-mail the study center with your questions.
- In the end, there are no guarantees of success, and it's impossible to know in advance which studies will be successful. To participate, you need to be fully informed and have confidence in the idea being tested and the research team involved.

7

Who Is Looking Out for You and What Can You Expect?

PERHAPS YOU HAVE QUESTIONS: "If I'm going to participate in a clinical trial, how will I know I'm going to be safe and protected? I signed a multipage consent form; does that mean I have *no* rights or legal recourse? What if I develop a life-threatening side effect? Who is looking out for me?" Read on for answers.

How Are Studies Overseen and Regulated?

Clinical trials are carefully monitored and overseen by many independent groups or committees, in addition to oversight by the pharmaceutical companies. At local institutions conducting studies—a hospital, academic center, or doctor's office—an institutional review board (IRB), more commonly known as an *ethics committee* (EC) outside of the United States, oversees clinical trials. The IRB's sole purpose is to ensure the protection of human subjects—that's you—as defined by federal laws and regulations. IRBs are local and independent, but federal law defines their responsibilities.

In the United States, the oversight of clinical trials at the federal level rests with the Office for Human Research Protections (OHRP). At the OHRP website www.hhs.gov/ohrp/, you can learn about the relevant regulations, policies, guidance, and rules under which IRBs are required to operate. The OHRP is responsible for educating researchers about the regulations and making sure they conduct their work "by the book." The OHRP carries the most authority. If an institution's IRB or investigators are not following the rules, the OHRP has the power to shut down all clinical research at that particular institution, and it has done just that—but only in rare instances.

When a clinical trial is stopped (a rare event), the best interest of the patients should always be the first priority. One possible scenario is that people in the trial can continue to receive treatment, but no new patients can join.

In large academic centers, clinical trials also undergo scrutiny by a scientific review committee. The IRB primarily focuses on patient safety, the quality of the consent form, and the accuracy and clarity of the information provided to the patient. The scientific review committee focuses on the scientific merit of proposed clinical trials. This extra step sometimes means that it takes longer to get a clinical trial under way at a large academic medical center than in a private practice setting. But it also means that more experts have reviewed it and, most likely, the study is of a high quality, scientifically well-designed, and asks an important question. These are the goals of the scientific review process.

The Power of the FDA

When a clinical trial involves a drug or a medical device, the U.S. Food and Drug Administration (FDA) provides another layer of oversight. Clinical trials must be submitted to the FDA with an Investigational New Drug (IND) application. This important document describes everything that is known to date about a drug, particularly the results of tests in animals and humans (if any have been done). All trials either have an IND number or they are considered IND exempt. IND-exempt studies are not sponsored by a pharmaceutical company, but instead are developed by independent researchers. These studies are not designed to gain approval for commercial sales of a drug, and they involve a drug that has been previously tested with similar patients. If a drug has only been tested in experimental animals, it must have an IND when first tested in humans.

Not One, but Two Animal Tests!

Before a person can take any drug, the FDA generally requires that it has first been tested in two animal species. The experience with these animals is vital to planning the human study. For example, the starting dose and side effects that need to be watched for are often determined by the animal studies. How a drug is metabolized (broken down internally) in the animals is also important in planning how it will be dosed in people. Drugs that are quickly eliminated from the body may need to be taken several times a day, or even given around the clock by intravenous infusion. Drugs that remain in the body for a longer period might be given once a day, once a week, or even once a month. The FDA requires regular reporting on the progress of clinical trials, especially with respect to adverse effects. It can withdraw approval for an IND if the clinical trial shows an unacceptable level of side effects, in which case the study must be stopped. If you want to learn more about the FDA's role in regulating clinical drug trials, you can go to: www.fda.gov/drugs/ developmentapprovalprocess/default.htm.

Truly Independent, All-Powerful Oversight: The Data Safety Monitoring Board

Phase III clinical trials—the large studies that compare one treatment to another—also have an independent data safety monitoring board (DSMB) or committee (DSMC). This is usually comprised of three or four scientists and statisticians who are completely independent of the researchers and the company. They have access to the unedited study data, and their job is to monitor progress and make sure that one arm of the study is not obviously better (or worse) than the other before the study is completed.

The DSMB looks at positive effects, such as cancer responses, longer survival, and cancer control—and negative results, such as side effects or worsening of the cancer. If the winner and loser become obvious early, the DSMB has the right—and the responsibility—to close the study and announce the results. One of the authors of this book (TMB) was involved in such a situation. Several studies of high-dose vitamin D in combination with chemotherapy yielded promising results, and a phase III randomized study was launched. Unfortunately, patients who got the high-dose vitamin D lived shorter lives than those who did not. While we still don't understand fully why this happened, the DSMB did its job and shut the study down early, notifying all the investigators and participants of their findings.

The DSMB is like a referee in a boxing match who has absolute authority to stop a fight early. If you are participating in a randomized study and are worried that you could be missing out on a better treatment, the DSMB is your "guardian angel." Its job is to make sure you know this kind of information as soon as anybody else does. Some studies have been closed suddenly and abruptly, much to the surprise of everyone involved. It can happen either because there were clear winners or clear losers.

If you are taking part in a clinical trial in a large health care system, such as the Department of Veterans Affairs (VA), or a large HMO such as Kaiser Permanente, there is probably another layer of oversight at the level of the organization. The VA, for example, has its own additional rules designed specifically to protect veterans.

The drug companies that sponsor trials and the senior or lead investigators involved in conducting them also carefully monitor clinical trials. They do a good job because they are solid professionals and, in no small measure, because they know that all the groups and boards discussed above are looking over their shoulders. Everybody wants to get it right. *You* want them to get it right, too. No area of your medical care will ever be as closely monitored as a clinical trial.

No area of your medical care will ever be as closely monitored as a clinical trial.

What Can I Expect From My Doctor and Investigative Team?

You can expect to receive close attention by a team of professionals that is often larger than what you might normally encounter during routine care. In addition to your doctor, often a study nurse will be your first point of contact for questions about such things as how you are doing and side effects. There will also be a study coordinator/data manager. In some programs, participants interact with the study coordinator. In other trials, study coordinators work in the background, and you only meet the nurse and your doctor. Most study coordinators are not medically trained. They are responsible for scheduling and coordinating all of your tests and visits, and for collecting and tracking the study data, which will include such things as the doses of the study drug you took, side effects, and the status of your cancer. Although they may be quite interested in your side effects, they should not give you medical advice on how to manage them—giving medical advice is the responsibility of your doctor and nurse.

You can expect exceptional care from the whole team, and you will almost certainly get more medical attention than if you were receiving standard care. You should also get regular reports about your progress. If you don't—*ask*! You're getting treatment for your cancer *and* you're helping the investigators. You are a *partner* in the trial. Be sure to ask, early on, for the name of the person to contact about specific concerns. Who should you call if you have a question about a scheduling matter, and who should you call if you are not feeling well, have a possible new side effect, or if you have a medical question? Having this information clarified from the start, and having all the right contact information for your research team, can go a long way toward making the process run smoothly and comfortably.

What If I Have Concerns and I'm Not Sure Where to Go for an Answer?

When in doubt, talk to your study doctor first—he is *always* the person in charge. The nurse is usually the best person to talk to about your medical concerns, and you can contact the study coordinator about scheduling and tests. They all have your interests at heart, and they want your experience in the trial to be a good one. Ask questions, share concerns, and note side effects.

Hopefully, this is all you will need, but if you think you are not getting the answers you expect or the service you deserve, look carefully at the copy of the consent form you signed. There is always a phone number for the head investigator, as well as for the IRB official who is responsible for oversight of the trial. These people are there for you, too!

Am I Free to Quit If I Want To?

Although you agreed to participate, you *always* have the right to quit. Your reasons might include side effects, not being comfortable with the trial, or other difficulties related to your care. Talk to your doctor and your trial team before you decide to leave. They may be able to resolve your concerns and answer your questions, so that you will be able to stay in the program. Cancer treatments, whether standard or investigational, can have unpleasant side effects. Sometimes, the simple adjustment of a dose of one of your medications, or an adjustment in your overall medication profile, might improve things and allow you to continue in the study.

You always retain the right to withdraw from a study at any time. When you sign up, you agree to start the trial, but you do not give up your right to change your mind.

You always retain the right to withdraw at any time. When you sign up, you agree to start the trial, but you do not give up your right to change your mind. If you decide to leave the study, it is important to be open about that with your research team and do it in collaboration with them. Some medications should not be stopped abruptly and some medication take days or even weeks to clear out of your body. Discontinuing treatment safely requires the advice and support of the research team and especially the doctor who is responsible for the study.

What If I Have Side Effects? How Will I Know If I Should Be Concerned?

Any new physical or emotional sensation that is out of the ordinary for you could be an adverse effect of the study drug. Tell the nurse and doctor about it. Your research team should explain to you when and how they want to hear from you about any new or more intense side effects you might experience. It is better to tell them sooner rather than later. There may be ways to manage your side effects. The problem may also turn out to be unrelated to the trial and might be treated separately while you continue in the trial. A few key principles:

- Always let the research team know about any changes in how you feel. Even if you have told your primary doctor or non-research health care personnel about any problems that develop, be sure to also tell the research team.
- Don't make changes in your medications or stop the study medication without talking to your research team—unless you are in an emergency situation, in which case you should take whatever action is necessary to manage the emergency and then contact the research team as soon a possible.

All of this is important, because an adverse effect caused by an experimental drug is different from ordinary side effects, mainly because less is known about it. A drug effect could start out mild and get worse over time if not addressed. Sometimes, this can happen very quickly. A primary care doctor who is not involved in research may not be familiar with the side effects of experimental medications and may not be as able to help you. The research team has access to a lot more information about the drug you are taking. In addition, any suspected side effect needs to be reported, so that all the other investigators and the oversight organizations and committees know about it. This does not mean that side effects from experimental therapies are necessarily serious, but they need to be brought to the attention of the research team promptly, so that they can be evaluated.

What If Something Goes Wrong?

The consent form you read and sign before you join a clinical trial will outline your rights. You are always entitled to attentive, thoughtful, and top-quality medical care to treat any side effect you experience. Some trials have a provision that the pharmaceutical company may cover the costs of your care for any complications from the experimental medication. Government-supported or institutional clinical trials don't offer such compensation. In most cases, you should expect your health insurance to be the primary source of coverage for your care while you are in a clinical trial, but always read the consent form carefully. If you are receiving care for an adverse effect of an experimental drug, you may be able to get these costs covered. Don't expect any compensation, however, for time lost, suffering, or any other personal difficulties. When you consent to participate in an investigational cancer treatment, there is an expectation that you may experience some side effects.

If negligence or malpractice is involved, you always have the right to ask an attorney for help, but thankfully these situations are rare.

How Do You Get Through the Red Tape?

At times, you may feel that the process of getting started on a clinical trial seems endless. Even when you have found the right trial for you, and it is open and actively seeking participants, weeks may pass, so that your current medications can be eliminated from your system. You will also be learning about the study, providing consent, completing the required tests, and scheduling your first treatment visit.

Read the consent form carefully before you sign it, and remember, you are always entitled to attentive, thoughtful, and top-quality medical care to treat any side effect you experience.

Spend this time reading everything carefully and asking questions to clarify anything you don't understand. Be persistent in advocating for yourself! If you are not getting the answers you need from one person, ask to be put in contact with someone who *can* answer your questions. The entire process works much better and faster when you are actively involved.

Why Are There Delays?

Most of the time, if a trial is a good fit for you and you are a good match for the trial, treatment will begin within several weeks or even sooner, but occasionally you will encounter delays. If you are facing delays, it is helpful to understand what is causing them.

Hopefully, the trial you are interested in is already open and active. If you are waiting for a study to start, the time to activation can vary quite a bit, depending on the review processes that trials must go through. Sometimes, contract negotiations between the medical facility and the pharmaceutical company can be delayed. If you are waiting for a trial to open, ask for an honest appraisal of where the trial stands in the activation process and how long it might take. Things are likely to move a bit faster or slower than everyone expects. If time is critical and delays are looming, consider all your options, including a different trial and starting or continuing standard treatments.

A trial that is up and running can also encounter delays. Sometimes, this is by design; for example, there is a built-in break in a phase I trial after the first few patients have received a particular dose to make sure no unexpected *toxicity* (serious side effect) exists. In these trials, there is usually a mandatory pause of about a month between groups starting treatment. If you are participating in a phase II trial, there may be a built-in pause after about half the patients have started. During this time, the investigators will review the effects of the treatment on the group. The study may be halted at this point if the early results are not sufficiently promising. These types of breaks are scheduled to protect you from receiving a treatment that may be overly toxic or ineffective.

Delays can also occur when the rationale and design of the study need to be reviewed and reconsidered. This can happen if unexpected side effects come to light, or if another effective treatment is developed. Rarely, delays can occur when the manufacturer falls behind in making sufficient supplies of the new drug for the study. Hopefully, you will not encounter undue delays, but if you do, understanding what you are up against will help you make sound decisions about what is best for you.

If the delay is clearly defined and you know what to expect—for example, you are told: "You will be able to start the trial treatment when 30 days have passed since your last standard treatment"—this may be manageable, and not too much different from the break that is often required between two standard treatments, such as chemotherapy and radiation. If the delay is open-ended and might become extended, you may wish to look for other clinical trials or treatment options. Open and honest communication with your research team is important.

Open and honest communication with your research team is important.

A Concern You May Have: "If I Start a Clinical Trial, and the Trial Medications Don't Work, I Could Be Wasting Valuable Time."

This is a common concern for both standard and experimental treatment. Almost all cancer treatments today are given for a period of time, and then an assessment is made to determine if they are working. This could be a scan, a blood test, a medical examination, or a pain survey, but some assessment to decide if a treatment is worth continuing is a routine part of cancer care.

A Misconception You May Encounter

"Doctors and hospitals make money on clinical trials, and as a result they have an incentive to produce positive results."

In most cases, hospitals and doctors *are* compensated for conducting studies. These clinical trials, however, are usually not a source of profit. The dollars from the sponsor primarily cover the salaries of the people who coordinate and run the trials. At most (if not all) academic medical centers, clinical research barely breaks even, or it might even lose money. This is, in part, because there are many government-sponsored studies for which the grants are too small to cover the costs, and institutional studies are often underfunded or even unfunded.

Strong safeguards are in place to ensure the integrity of the clinical trial process. Lead investigators on clinical trials are prohibited from owning stock, working for, or consulting for the companies that own and manufacture the drug. The scientists who interpret the results should have no incentive to make the study turn out one way or another. The FDA oversees pharmaceutical companies, and it can—and does—audit studies to make sure the results are reported accurately. Fake results and fraud are exceedingly rare in clinical research.

A Misconception You May Encounter

"Most clinical trials carefully pick the patients with the least serious types and levels of cancer, in order to improve the chances for success."

Cancer treatment drugs are developed for all levels and stages of cancer. Participants need to meet certain criteria, so that any results will be relevant and the trial process can be as short as possible. There is no question, however, that many trials exclude the sickest patients, particularly those whose heart, lungs, kidneys, or liver are not working very well. This is done to protect patients. We don't know a lot about the safety of new drugs. Patients with liver or kidney problems are particularly susceptible to drug toxicity, and they need to be healthy enough to recover from any side effects. After a drug is approved for patients who are relatively healthy, additional studies may be done to make sure that we can safely give the drug to others whose health is not quite as good.

Clinical trials are no different. Each clinical trial comes with a specific plan that defines how long the treatment will be given and how your cancer will be monitored. Ask about this before you start, and also ask specifically about how long your cancer might be allowed to progress before your treatment is changed. Often, you will find out that it is not any longer than it would be with standard treatment. Sometimes, it may be longer because the study criteria are more stringent than routine care. Understand this and make sure you are comfortable with the treatment plan the study proposes. Remember that trial designs must also be judged ethical. Letting your cancer grow unchecked for a prolonged period of time would not be ethical in most situations and would not be desirable for anyone. Trials should be designed to monitor the status of your cancer thoroughly and to consider other treatments when they would be medically beneficial. Finally, if you are comfortable with the trial design when you enter a study—but you change your mind later—remember, you can stop participating at any time.

THE BOTTOM LINE

- Seek the support of your oncologist, your primary care doctor, your spouse, and others around you while you are making decisions about whether to sign up for a study and also while you are participating in the trial.
- Clinical trials are tightly regulated and closely supervised by the study team, institutional committees, independent boards, pharmaceutical companies, and the government. The scrutiny is far more extensive than what you would receive during routine cancer care.
- Most of your medical care will be billed to and covered by your health insurance company while you're participating in a study. Items that are purely for research are generally provided free of charge.
- It is important to establish and maintain clear communication with your entire study team:
  - Find out which members of the team are the right contacts for different types of questions and concerns.
  - Let your study team know about any adverse effects (side effects) or concerns promptly.
  - Don't try to solve problems that arise on your own or wait until your next appointment—contact your team whenever any difficulty arises.
- You are always free to stop being a part of a study. If you are thinking about stopping, be frank with your doctor and research team. You may learn that they can solve your problems or address your concerns without stopping the study treatment.
- If you encounter delays, find out the reasons for them, understand how long they may take, and do what is best for your health. If time is critical, consider all of your options.

8

Who Pays for Clinical Trials—And What Can They Cost?

HOW EXPENSIVE COULD PARTICIPATING in a clinical trial be, you ask? Quite expensive actually—for someone—but usually not for you.* From the earliest laboratory experiments through the many phases of trials, and ultimately the U.S. Food and Drug Administration (FDA) approval process, the total cost to develop a new drug can be well into the tens or even hundreds of millions of dollars! This is a major reason why new drugs are so expensive. It is not uncommon for the newest and most effective drugs to cost $1,000, $2,000, or even $5,000 or more each month, but you're probably well aware of this already. Your health insurance and drug coverage may pay most, some, or none of these costs. You'll want to check this out before beginning any new chemotherapy or other drug treatment. As you may know, medical costs are a leading cause of bankruptcies in the United States, and this risk increases as you get older, although Medicare is usually supportive of cancer care.

From the beginning, the drug company sponsoring a clinical trial is taking a gamble. It is betting its time, expertise, and money that a new drug will be effective and that the company will get its investment back—and make a profit, too. However, many experimental drugs fail

*Health insurance and health care costs vary a great deal around the world. In this chapter we describe the current situation in the United States. If you live elsewhere, we would encourage you to discuss these issues with your doctor, your health insurance provider, and local support groups.

to receive FDA approval, and the drug companies can lose millions in the process. As a result, successful drugs not only have to earn their own costs back, but they also need to earn enough to pay the costs of all the drugs that did not make it through the approval process.

What Costs Are Involved in Clinical Trials?

When you think about the costs of a clinical trial, you will probably focus on the costs of your own care, called *clinical care costs.* This includes such things as laboratory tests and scans. As expensive as these may be, they actually represent only a fraction of the total costs of a study. The salaries of the people who make clinical trials a reality are the largest expense. You are likely to work directly with study coordinators, study nurses, and investigators. In addition, there are many people working in clinical trials you will likely not deal with directly: pharmacists, the laboratory technicians who handle your blood specimens, the regulatory specialists who make sure the trial has all the necessary approvals (see Chapter 7), and all the people who oversee the clinical trial process to make sure it is being done correctly. These are just the people who work at the one hospital or research center you are visiting—they are only the "tip of the iceberg."

A large group of people at the pharmaceutical company, or subcontracted by it, develop the study procedures; receive, review, and analyze the results; monitor all side effects; disseminate information to all the researchers (for example, new serious side effect information has to be circulated right away to everyone involved); and interact with the FDA. This army of people behind any clinical trial can cost a small—or even a large—fortune!

Who Pays for These Costs?

This is an interesting question, but you probably care more about the clinical care costs that will affect *you.* In general, items that are solely for research, such as the study drug and highly specialized tests that would not otherwise be done to take care of you and treat your cancer, are covered by the study budget. They are free to you. All of the other costs of medical care—which you would generally expect to need even if you were not in a clinical trial—are billed to you and your health insurance company.

All the other costs of running a clinical trial are borne by the pharmaceutical company sponsoring the study. However, not all studies have an industry sponsor. Some research ideas, although important, are unlikely to be tested by a pharmaceutical company. For example, if we discover that a commonly used drug that is available as a *generic* could have a beneficial use in cancer therapy, a pharmaceutical company is almost never willing to get involved. *Generic* is the term used for a less expensive version of a brand-name drug that becomes available after the brand-name version goes *off-patent*, meaning the patent has expired. The lack of patent protection and the inexpensive cost of generic drugs make this type of research a poor business proposition.

Such studies are typically designed and led by individual researchers who must find the funding to support them. Sometimes, this involves a grant from the pharmaceutical industry, a grant from a federal government source (most commonly the National Cancer Institute [NCI] or Department of Defense), or a grant from a private organization, such as the American Cancer Society (ACS). Philanthropic donors or the hospital itself fund some studies. Some studies have no funding at all, and the investigating team donates their time. Although university administrators frown on unfunded studies because the people involved still get their salaries from the university, academic professors can be quite innovative about making these trials happen when they are truly excited about a new idea.

Costs of Your Care and Insurance Coverage of Cancer Clinical Trials

Misconceptions and concerns about health care costs during cancer clinical trials are common. Some patients, and some doctors, think that experimental treatment is always free. *This is almost never true.* Some studies do provide all of the care for free, but in the world of cancer research, these are more often the exception than the rule.

Most completely free studies are pure experiments, not actual efforts to treat cancer. An example would be a study that gives you a single dose of a brand new drug that has never been taken by a human being and then collects blood samples to determine how quickly the body breaks down the new drug. With a single dose, you would hardly expect that your cancer would be affected in the slightest. Such studies lack what is called *therapeutic intent*—they are an experiment and not a treatment. These studies are often conducted in healthy volunteers rather than in people with cancer. In addition to providing care for free, many also provide some compensation for the time and risks involved. If you have cancer and are looking for a treatment to help you fight it, a one-time experimental study is *not* for you.

For studies designed to *treat* cancer, your health insurance will be billed for many elements of your care. This type of study usually provides—free of charge—any unapproved drugs and the things that are done purely to learn about the drug rather than take care of you, such as blood draws to measure drug levels. As noted above, everything that would happen normally if you were getting a standard treatment, including physician visits, routine blood tests, routine scans, and other tests needed to monitor your health, are typically billed to your insurance. This is always spelled out in the consent form, but it may be difficult to sort out. Check the fine print and ask a health professional for help if it seems confusing.

Is your health insurance willing to pay? If so, how much? Is there a chance you will get stuck with the bill? It could happen, but much can be done to prevent it if you are proactive. We believe that until all patients with cancer can expect a reliable cure, well-designed clinical trials should be part of *standard care.* Unfortunately, no single answer applies to every person with cancer. Read on to learn how you can make sure that no financial surprises are present in your clinical trial.

Medicare Comes Through

If you are over the age of 65, chances are Medicare is part—or even all—of your health care coverage. Many insurance companies, to some extent, follow the approach Medicare takes in deciding what it will cover and what it won't. So, even if you don't yet have Medicare, it's worth understanding the rules for Medicare recipients.

Since 2000, Medicare has covered the *routine costs of qualifying clinical trials.* In addition, it covers the costs of diagnosing and caring for complications arising from participation in all qualifying clinical trials. As with all legal matters, it is worth understanding the key definitions involved in this.

Routine costs are those items and services that are generally available to all Medicare beneficiaries (who signed up for Part B, for which a premium is paid monthly). This includes doctor visits, routine laboratory tests, scans, and tests needed to monitor your condition. Medicare also covers the costs associated with giving the experimental agent. This is not significant if the treatment is given in pill form, but costs can be high if it involves an intravenous infusion. So, it's always good to know exactly what is covered. If Medicare doesn't usually cover something, such as cosmetic surgery, it will not cover it while you are a part of a clinical trial. Medicare does not cover experimental drugs or devices, or items and services that are used solely to gather and analyze research data rather than to take care of you, such as blood drug levels or exploratory tests.

Most of the time, these definitions are understandable. One "gray area" is a situation in which something that is routinely done is required more frequently during the study than would be done ordinarily. Let's say a study requires a computed tomography (CT) scan twice a year, but you would most likely only have one a year if you were not in a trial. This is a gray area because, in most cases, there is no absolute standard for how often patients need blood tests or scans when they are receiving care for cancer. Some situations require more frequent monitoring than others. Some doctors, and some patients, prefer more frequent monitoring than others. The *standard* is really a range in which doctors actually practice. Situations exist in which something that would ordinarily be considered quite routine is done so frequently in a study that Medicare won't cover it. Your research team and the institutional oversight committee (the Institutional Review Board or IRB, as discussed in Chapter 7) are expected to pay attention to these matters and identify situations for which Medicare or your insurance will not cover costs. In these situations, the trial sponsor would usually be expected to pay. You'll obviously want to know in advance if it's going to come out of your own pocket.

If you notice that the study you are considering requires frequent tests, check with the study team about the costs involved and who pays for them. Many institutions develop a *costs of care or clinical billing*

Sample Clinical Billing Schedule

Week	1	2	5	9	13	17
Standard Care Services (Billed to Insurance)						
Physical Exam	X	X	X	X	X	X
Vital Signs	X	X	X	X	X	X
CT or MRI Scan	X				X	
Bone Scan	X				X	
Routine Clinical Labs	X	X	X	X	X	X
Study-Related Services (Free to You; Paid For by the Study)						
Pharmacy: Study Drug Dispensing Fees	X		X	X	X	X
Pharmacy: Study Drug Storage	X	X	X	X	X	X
Special Labs	X	X	X	X	X	X
Drug Level Monitoring Sample	X	X	X	X	X	

CT, computed tomography; MRI, magnetic resonance imaging

schedule for each study. These tables spell out every planned item and service that is a part of the study, and they make it clear whether each item will be provided free of charge or billed to your insurance.

The second part of the Medicare requirement is that the study you are part of is a *qualifying study*. If you are at a reputable medical center that has experience with clinical research, nearly all studies are qualifying studies. Just to be sure, ask the study team if the prospective trial is qualified. The basic requirements are that the study involves a type of treatment that is ordinarily covered by Medicare (which cancer care is, of course) and that the study must have *therapeutic intent*—meaning that its goal is to treat your cancer. This is what you want—a study designed to treat cancer and not just test a drug's side effects or blood concentrations.

Finally, to qualify, the trials have to involve patients who have a disease, not healthy volunteers, unless a healthy volunteer group is needed as a control group for comparison to people with cancer.

These are the main requirements.

Additional characteristics that trials should have in order to qualify, all of which are generally sensible, include:

- They should have the goal of improving the lives of people with cancer.
- They should be well conceived and designed.
- They should be conducted with integrity.

Although some of these characteristics are a bit vague, they are all features that you would want in a trial. Medicare also presumes that many federally supported institutions would only conduct trials that meet these basic standards. As a result, trials supported by such institutions automatically qualify; for example, if you are considering a trial at a cancer center that has been designated as such by the NCI, or at a Veterans Administration (VA) hospital, the trials will automatically qualify for Medicare coverage.

The Medicare Loophole—Recently Closed, Thank Goodness!

Although Medicare covers routine costs for participants in clinical trials, until January 1, 2011, people who enrolled in a Medicare Advantage plan, rather than standard Medicare, discovered that the Advantage plans did not cover their copays during clinical trial participation. The only option for people in this situation was to have their care billed under traditional Medicare, which covered the trial but with invariably higher copayments. As one of the changes included in the Health Care Reform Law, starting January 1, 2011, Medicare Advantage plans are now required to cover copays for participants in clinical trials in the same way they would if the patient was not enrolled in a clinical trial. Health care regulations are always changing, and the Health Care Reform Law is being challenged in the courts and in Congress, so keep an eye on this issue and check with your plan before you start a clinical trial.

Traditional Health Insurance

No two health insurance plans are exactly alike. If your coverage is outside of Medicare, you will need to check what it covers. Your research team may do this for you by requesting preauthorization for care during a clinical trial. Ask them to do this if nobody mentions it. There is some risk that your insurer will deny approval, but it's worth inquiring, and you'll have peace of mind knowing you will be covered.

It Matters Where You Live

Health insurance is regulated by the individual states, for the most part. Many states have passed laws that require insurers to cover routine costs of care for participants in a clinical trial. As of November 2011, 34 states and Washington D.C. have laws or special agreements that govern this issue, but 16 states and Puerto Rico have not yet acted on it. New laws are being introduced in many parts of the country, so the number could be higher by the time you read this. Each law is unique, although the general idea of each may be similar to the principles used in developing Medicare's policy.

Health insurance is regulated by the individual states, for the most part. Many states have passed laws that require insurers to cover routine costs of care for participants in a clinical trial.

Several websites provide information about current laws. The American Cancer Society (ACS) maintains a list at: www.cancer.org/Treatment/TreatmentsandSideEffects/ClinicalTrials/StateLawsRegardingInsuranceCoverage/clinical-trials-state-laws-clin-trials-laws-by-state.

The NCI provides a map of states that have passed legislation on this matter and a summary of the provisions of each of the laws at: www.cancer.gov/clinicaltrials/payingfor/laws.

States that are darker gray on the map below have laws that address insurance coverage for participants in clinical trials.

If you live in a state that requires insurance plans to cover routine costs of care (in dark gray), chances are you'll have little difficulty with your health insurance company. Preauthorization and information

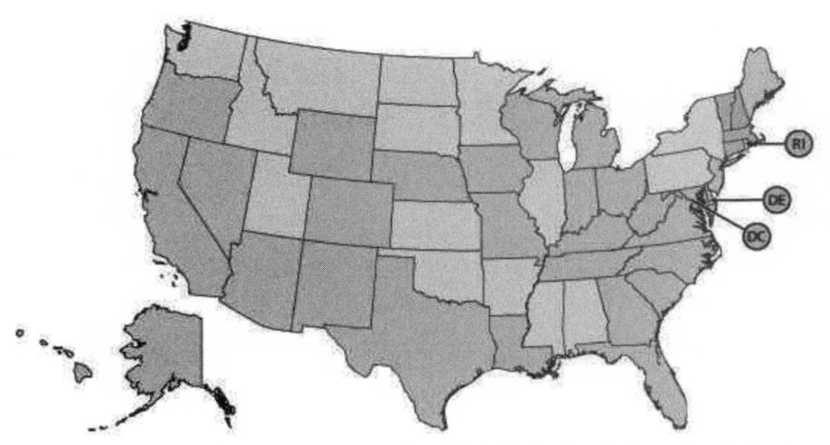

Insurance Coverage for Participants in Clinical Trials by State. States in dark gray require health plans to cover at least some patient care costs in clinical trials. Details of these requirements by state are available at www.cancer.gov/clinicaltrials/payingfor/laws. If you live in a state that does not have such a legal requirement, this does not mean that your insurer will not cover the costs associated with participation in a clinical trial. It simply means that there is no legal requirement to do so and insurers are free to decide how to handle these costs. Reprinted with permission, National Cancer Institute, updated as of November 25, 2011.

about the clinical trial may need to be sent to them before you start the clinical trial, particularly information that is relevant to making sure the clinical trial qualifies for coverage. Your research team will probably take care of this, but in some circumstances, you may need to get involved.

The Health Care Reform Act of 2010 also stipulates that routine costs for care of clinical trial participants will be covered nationwide. However, these provisions don't go into effect until January 1, 2014.

What If Your Health Insurer Denies Coverage?

If you receive a denial, don't give up! *Appeal!* It's not uncommon for an initial denial to be issued by a person who is not fully familiar with cancer clinical trials, and there is a good chance that the decision can be changed with additional information. Make sure you're prepared before you attempt to do this. You need to be armed with accurate information in order to win. First, talk to your doctor and your research team, and decide who will take the lead on an appeal. It may be helpful for you and your team to pursue it at the same time. It may depend on your insurer's procedures for appeal.

You will need to learn the following:

- What is the process for appealing a coverage denial decision with your insurer?
- How long should it take to receive a response from a regular appeal?
- What is the process for filing an emergency appeal? A regular appeal often takes several weeks, and you may not wish to let this much time go by. Anyone who is considering a new cancer therapy deserves a fast answer, so don't be bashful about making an emergency appeal. If too much time goes by, you could miss the window of opportunity for participating in the trial.
- What rules does your insurance company follow in determining whether routine costs of care are covered for participants in clinical trials? *This is the single most important question you need to ask.* An appeal is more likely to be successful if you have the facts on your side. If the company has a set of criteria, and the trial you are inter-

ested in meets the criteria, but they simply did not know or did not consider them, all you have to do is clearly articulate your case, point by point, and show that the trial meets their own criteria. One simple example would be a situation in which your insurance company follows Medicare guidelines. In this case, pointing out that the trial you are interested in meets all the requirements to be a *qualifying* trial under Medicare rules might be a sufficient argument.

- Does your plan have any exceptions for *life-threatening conditions* that may allow you to circumvent any restrictions? Cancer is often a life-threatening condition, and you should not hesitate to point this out if the company has such an exception.

Armed with this information, you and/or your doctor should file a written appeal and follow-up to make sure it gets the attention it deserves. Sometimes, a phone call from your doctor directly to the insurance company's medical director can break through the log-jam. If your doctor does not offer, don't be afraid to suggest it. A sample appeal letter is shown on the next page. Obviously, it needs to be adapted to your personal circumstances to make certain that all the statements you make in the letter are clear, concise, true, and accurate.

Other Approaches

If an appeal and phone call from your doctor doesn't work, you may still have other options. If you live in a state in which the law requires coverage, and you feel that your insurer is not complying with the law, you may wish to ask for help from the state office that oversees insurers. It might also be useful to contact your local state senator and/or representative. This can be particularly helpful if they contributed to passing the law, as they may be eager to see it implemented to help their constituents. Your local newspaper or radio or TV station may have a consumer help desk or service. Like all businesses, insurance companies don't like negative attention from legislators or the media. Don't hesitate to "pull out all the stops."

Sample appeal letter from a doctor's office*

DATE

To: *YOUR INSURANCE COMPANY APPEALS DEPARTMENT*

RE: Emergency Appeal of Coverage Denial for *YOUR NAME*

Medical Record Number:

Insurance ID Number:

Reference Case Number:
(this number may be provided in the denial letter)

Date of Birth:

Mr./Ms. *YOUR NAME* has advanced cancer of ___________ and wishes to receive an investigational therapy, using the agent ___________ while participating in a National Cancer Institute approved clinical trial (NCI PDQ Number ___________, Institutional Review Board Number___________).

The following recounts the events that preceded this appeals letter:

On *DATE* our office faxed to *INSURANCE COMPANY* on behalf of my patient *YOUR NAME* a request for authorization for coverage of *standard of care costs* pursuant to this clinical trial. These costs include routine physician visits, routine laboratory tests, and computed tomography (CT) and bone scans *(MAKE SURE THIS LIST IS ACCURATE FOR YOUR TRIAL)*. *It is important to note that all of these procedures represent routine staging and monitoring of cancer.* The cost and coverage of the drug itself is provided at no cost and is not included in this request. Authorization for these services was denied by *NAME OF THE PERSON*, who signed the denial letter on *DATE*. It is important to note several essential points about this clinical trial

(*CHOOSE THOSE THAT APPLY TO YOU*):

- The trial is fully approved by the Food and Drug Administration and *ANY OTHER RELEVANT AGENCY OR ORGANIZATION* and is being carried out at an NCI-designated cancer center (*IF TRUE*).
- The trial meets all stipulations of CMS (Medicare) guidance regarding coverage of routine care for patients enrolled in clinical trials. Most insurance companies follow these federal guidelines regarding coverage decisions.

- Coverage for routine costs of care for patients enrolled in this and similar clinical trials is required by law in the State of *YOUR STATE (IF YOU RESIDE IN A STATE WITH LAWS REGARDING INSURANCE COVERAGE)*.
- The trial meets all criteria for required for coverage under your policy. Specifically, it meets the following criteria (*BE SPECIFIC AND COMPLETE IF YOU HAVE DISCOVERED THAT YOUR INSURER HAS CRITERIA AND THAT YOUR TRIAL MEETS THEM*).

YOUR NAME has an unambiguously life-threatening cancer for which no standard curative therapy is available. The only available therapy that remains for him/her is ____________ (*FILL IN THE BLANK*), which offers limited benefits at significant costs. OR No standard therapy is available for him/her.

Insurance companies frequently have exceptions to their coverage restrictions specifically for life-threatening conditions and treatments not available within the plan. This is clearly such a case, and coverage should be provided.

The study provides the investigational drug. Thus, the costs of care on the clinical trial are likely to be less than if the treatment consisted of standard chemotherapy (*OR WHATEVER IS THE ALTERNATIVE*) outside of a clinical trial.

Denial of coverage would force *YOUR NAME* to be treated with potentially toxic and marginally effective chemotherapy at a greater cost. This would not serve the patient, the insurance company, or society.

I therefore ask that you expeditiously consider this request for coverage. Because *YOUR NAME* has an incurable cancer, I request that this appeal be considered as an emergency appeal. I will be pleased to provide any additional information you may require.

Respectfully yours,

PHYSICIAN'S NAME, MD

**Can be adapted to come from the patient as well*

But There's More

There is one exception to the rules we've discussed so far. Although most health insurance is regulated by the states, many large employers are *self-insured.* Most people who work for self-insured companies don't even know it, because their insurance functions just like regular insurance. The company hires a traditional insurance firm to administer the health plan and carry out functions, such as claims processing, payment, and claim denials. The difference behind the scenes is that the financial risk is borne by the large employer rather than the insurance company. Insurance companies make a profit from taking on risk, so self-insurance can save your employer money, provided the organization is large enough to absorb the risk.

Although most health insurance is regulated by the states, many large employers are self-insured.

Self-insurance is primarily regulated by the federal Employee Retirement Income Security Act (ERISA) and not by state insurance regulators. State laws that mandate insurance coverage for routine costs of

A Misconception You May Encounter

"Most clinical trials claim to be free, but hidden costs can add up to many thousands of dollars, and most health insurance plans won't cover them."

Most clinical trials are not totally free and do not claim to be. Parts of the study are generally provided free of charge, including the investigational medication and tests that are done solely for the experiment and not to take care of your medical needs. Ongoing care for your cancer is often billed to you and your insurance provider. Many insurance providers cover such expenses. Each trial is different, and all of this information should be spelled out in the consent form. Read it carefully and *ask questions.*

care may not apply to self-insurance health plans. This does not necessarily mean that such plans will deny coverage. Many self-insured organizations recognize the importance of access to clinical trials for their employees. It just means that you may have one less lever to use in an appeal if you do receive a denial. The ERISA law does not address clinical trials, and any changes that would require ERISA-regulated health plans to cover clinical trials would need to occur at the federal level.

The Bottom Line

- Until standard cancer therapy is much more effective and reliable cancer cures are common, participation in clinical trials should be an option for nearly everyone with cancer.
- Medicare covers the routine costs of care for recipients who participate in qualified clinical trials. The investigational drugs or devices themselves and procedures that are purely for research purposes (not designed for your ongoing medical care) are not covered. Services that would not normally be covered under Medicare are not covered.
- Many insurers have policies that provide for similar coverage, but this varies from plan to plan and state to state.
- The majority of states have passed laws that require coverage for clinical trial participants.
- The Health Care Reform Act of 2010 requires all health plans to cover clinical trials by January 1, 2014.
- Large companies that are self-insured are regulated by the federal ERISA law and may not be impacted by state laws. ERISA does not address clinical trials.
- Your research team should communicate with your insurer to gain approval for your coverage before you begin participation.
- If you are denied coverage, work with your doctor and research team to appeal. An appeal based on knowledge of your insurer's

policies, your state's laws, and the particulars regarding the trial in which you are interested has the best chance of success. A call from your doctor to your insurance company's medical director can also be helpful.

Part IV

Medical Treatment of Cancer Now and in the Future

9

Cancer Drugs Currently in Use and Being Tested in Trials

The list of new drugs being studied in clinical trials changes frequently. We will keep you updated on our blog at: www.cancer-clinical-trials.com/.

THE DEVELOPMENT OF ANTICANCER DRUGS began in earnest in the 1940s. Today, hundreds of them are in standard use and in clinical trials. Even more are still in development. The list changes frequently—an indicator of the progress being made. We won't provide an exhaustive list, but instead tell you about *drug families*—groups of drugs that work in similar ways—and provide examples of each. As you navigate the world of cancer therapy and clinical trials, you may find that the drug being offered to you belongs to one of these categories. We will first give the generic name where it exists, with the brand names in parentheses, where they exist. Some drugs have multiple brand names.

CHEMOTHERAPY DRUGS

There are many subcategories of chemotherapy drugs, and they are identified by the mechanism through which they kill cancer cells.

Because these drugs have to be taken at high doses, normal tissues can't completely escape damage. This is what causes the commonly experienced side effects of chemotherapy.

Chemotherapy side effects vary considerably between classes of chemotherapy drugs, as well as between individual drugs. They also vary considerably among individuals. It is not uncommon for one person to have a difficult time, while another experiences few or no problems, despite the fact that both are receiving the same dose of the same drug.

Cancer cells grow more rapidly than most normal cells, and chemotherapy attacks the mechanisms that cause rapid cell growth. As a consequence, the most common chemotherapy side effects are related to the effects of these drugs on the normally rapidly dividing cells in our bodies, such as infection-fighting white cells, oxygen-carrying red cells, and the platelets responsible for blood clotting. Blood cells have a limited lifespan, and new ones are continually replenishing those that have died. Hair grows continually under normal conditions, and a common effect of chemotherapy is to decrease hair growth and cause hair loss. Similarly, the lining of our entire gastrointestinal tract is made up of cells that are continuously replaced. For this reason, mouth sores, upset stomach, and diarrhea are not uncommon with chemotherapy.

Nausea is another common side effect of chemotherapy. The nausea caused by chemotherapy is generally not an effect on the actual stomach or intestines, but rather a direct effect on the brain. This knowledge has led to the development of effective antinausea drugs that have considerably reduced the impact of this side effect.

Some, but not all, chemotherapy drugs can cause *peripheral neuropathy*—damage to nerves that causes numbness, tingling, and loss of sensation. These symptoms may gradually disappear when chemotherapy is stopped, but in some cases they are permanent.

Many chemotherapy drugs cause fatigue, particularly when given over a period of several months. This common problem can be improved somewhat with regular exercise, but there is no foolproof solution for it. You need to allow for this, and accept that there may be days when you do not have the energy to do much at all.

In addition to these common side effects, each chemotherapy drug has its own unique side-effect profile. All patients receiving chemotherapy, whether or not a clinical trial is involved, should be familiar with the common risks and side effects, and communicate with the care team if they experience any. Many side effects can be counteracted with additional medications or reduced when the dose of chemotherapy is lowered slightly.

The nausea caused by chemotherapy is generally not an effect on the actual stomach or intestines, but rather a direct effect on the brain. This knowledge has led to the development of effective antinausea drugs that have considerably reduced the impact of this side effect.

Antimetabolites

Antimetabolites were among the first chemotherapy agents. As is common to many types of chemotherapeutic agents, they interfere with the production of DNA and RNA. DNA is our master genetic code. It contains all of our genes and requires duplication of the entire DNA code during *cell division*, when a cell divides into two new ones. RNA is produced continuously in cells. Its functions include transmitting the information encoded in DNA to make the proteins that are the key building blocks of the human cell, and it serves other key functions within these cells.

DNA and RNA production occurs in essentially all cells of the body, so these drugs are not cancer-specific. They take advantage of the fact that cancer cells divide more often than most normal cells and are often less able to repair DNA or RNA damage than normal cells.

Examples of antimetabolites include 5-fluorouracil (5-FU), capecitabine (Xeloda®), 6-mercaptopurine (6-MP), methotrexate, gemcitabine (Gemzar®), cytarabine (Ara-C®), fludarabine (Fludara®), and pemetrexed (Alimta®).

Alkylating Agents

In some ways that are similar to the effects of radiation therapy, *alkylating agents* damage the DNA itself, which makes successful cell division more difficult. Like many chemotherapeutic agents, this family of drugs relies on the fact that normal cells can handle the damage and make repairs better than cancer cells can, although this repair capacity is not perfect. The first alkylating agent was developed after the observation that the deadly World War I chemical weapon called *mustard gas* caused lymph nodes to shrink.

There are many subclasses of alkylating agents, including the nitrogen mustards: nitrogen mustard (Mustargen®), chlorambucil (Leukeran®), melphalan (Alkeran®), cyclophosphamide (Cytoxan®), ifosfamide (Ifex®); and the nitrosoureas: streptozocin (Zanosar®), carmustine (BiCNU®, Gliadel®), and lomustine (CeeNU®).

Alkylating agents that are not based on nitrogen mustard include busulfan (Busulfex®), dacarbazine (DTIC®, DTIC-Dome®), temozolomide (Temodar®), thiotepa (Tioplex®), and hexamethylmelamine (Hexalen®).

DNA Cross-Linking Platinum Derivatives

These drugs are similar to alkylating agents in that they damage DNA. This category of drugs was discovered in 1965 by a stroke of luck, when a platinum electrode in a laboratory dish unexpectedly caused nearby *Escherichia coli* bacteria to stop growing. Subsequent experiments confirmed similar effects against cancer cells. The first drug of this type, cisplatin, was approved in 1978. Cisplatin is a derivative of platinum that has made the cure of testicular cancer not only possible, but also nearly routine.

In addition to cisplatin (Platinol®), this drug family includes carboplatin (Paraplatin®), oxaliplatin (Eloxatin®), and the investigational agents satraplatin and picoplatin.

Antitumor Antibiotics

These agents interfere with the enzymes that duplicate our DNA, an essential step in cell division.

This class of drugs, the anthracycline group of antibiotics, includes daunorubicin (Cerubidine®), doxorubicin (Adriamycin®), epirubicin (Ellence®), and idarubicin (Idamycin PFS®). Other examples of antitumor antibiotics include actinomycin-D (Cosmegen®), bleomycin (Blenoxane®), mitomycin-C (Mutamycin®), and mitoxantrone (Novantrone®).

Topoisomerase Inhibitors

These drugs interfere with specific enzymes that help unwind a cell's DNA, which is a necessary step in its duplication. Topotecan (Hycamtin®), irinotecan (Camptosar®), etoposide (Vepesid®), and teniposide (Vumon®) belong to this class of agents.

Microtubule Assembly and Disassembly Inhibitors (Mitotic Inhibitors)

Microtubules are relatively rigid structures inside a human cell that provide the physical scaffolding that organizes cell division. When microtubules do not function properly, cell division often fails and the cell dies. A number of drugs interfere with microtubules by stopping their ability to assemble or disassemble. Either approach can work, because microtubules are formed from tiny pieces of protein that must come together and come apart frequently.

There are several subcategories of these drugs, including:

- Taxanes: paclitaxel (Taxol® or Abraxane®), docetaxel (Taxotere®), and cabazitaxel (Jevtana®), as well as the investigational drug xyotax (Opaxio®)
- Epothilones: ixabepilone (Ixempra®)

- Vinca alkaloids: vinblastine (Velban®), vincristine (Oncovin®), and vinorelbine (Navelbine®)
- Nontaxane halichondrin B analog microtubule inhibitors: eribulin mesylate (Halaven®)

Chemotherapy is the largest and best-known category of anticancer drugs, but there are also many other important drug categories, as discussed below.

Hormonal Agents

This class of drugs usually lowers or blocks the activity of specific hormones. For example, breast and prostate cancers are frequently dependent on hormones for their growth, and, thus, hormonal therapies can be effective in treating these cancers.

Testosterone- and Estrogen-Lowering Drugs

The original way to get rid of the sex hormones—testosterone and estrogen—was to surgically remove the main sources of production: the testicles in men and the ovaries in women. Drugs were developed to block the action of hormones and make surgery unnecessary. They do this through several different mechanisms.

Pituitary Gland-Based Drugs

Leuprolide acetate (Lupron®, Eligard®) and goserelin acetate (Zoladex®) suppress signals from the pituitary gland, the master gland in the brain that tells the testicles and ovaries to produce hormones.

Degarelix (Firmagon®) does essentially the same thing, but avoids the initial rise in hormones that can occur during the first weeks of therapy with drugs in the leuprolide category.

Testosterone Production-Lowering Drugs

Abiraterone acetate (Zytiga®) and TAK-700 suppress the enzymes that synthesize hormones and are used to treat prostate cancer. Ketoconazole, an anti-fungal antibiotic, has also been used as a hormone lowering agent for many years although it was neither designed for this purpose nor approved by the FDA for this indication. These enzymes are activated by signals from the pituitary, but they can also be turned on inappropriately in cancer. When this happens, the cancer essentially drives its own growth. Drugs in this category can counteract these growth signals.

Estrogen Production-Lowering Drugs

Anastrazole (Arimidex®), letrozole (Femara®), and similar drugs suppress the enzymes that synthesize estrogen.

Hormone-Blocking Drugs

Unlike drugs that decrease the production of hormones, hormone-blocking drugs compete with natural hormones for access to hormone receptors. This is the main mechanism through which hormones exert their influence on cells, including cancer cells. When they bind to the receptor—instead of activating it as the hormone would—hormone-blocking drugs block the ability of hormones to act. If you think of hormones as the key and receptors the lock, hormone blockers take the key's place in the lock, so it can't be used. Hormone blockers are therefore able to block the action of hormones even if they are still present. This avoids the necessity of surgically removing hormone-producing tissue. This class of drugs includes both testosterone and estrogen blockers.

Hormone-blocking drugs compete with natural hormones for access to hormone receptors. This is the main mechanism through which hormones exert their influence on cells, including cancer cells. The use of these drugs avoids the necessity of surgically removing the testicles in men and the ovaries in women.

Testosterone-blocking drugs include bicalutamide (Casodex®), flutamide (Eulexin®), and nilutamide (Nilandron®). These drugs are approved *androgen receptor blockers*—androgen receptors are the same as *testosterone receptors.* MDV-3100 is an experimental drug that may be a more potent drug in this category.

Estrogen-blocking drugs are similar to testosterone blockers. They bind to the estrogen receptor, block it, and keep naturally occurring estrogen from stimulating cancer cells. Examples include tamoxifen (Nolvadex®), raloxifene (Evista®), and toremifene (Fareston®). Fulvestrant (Faslodex®) has a similar effect, but its mechanism is somewhat distinct. Instead of binding to estrogen receptors, it reduces the number of these receptors in cancer cells.

Testosterone Conversion/Activation Blockers

To be fully active, testosterone must first be converted to *dihydrotestosterone* (DHT). Drugs in this category block this activation step. Examples include finasteride (Proscar®) and dutasteride (Avodart®).

Small-Molecule Targeted Drugs

These are custom-designed modern cancer drugs that seek to interfere with specific aspects of cancer cells. Often taken by mouth, these drugs represent the latest advances in cancer therapy. In some cases, they work well on their own. In other situations, they are combined with chemotherapy. These drugs are also sometimes also referred to as *biologic therapy*. They include:

- **Imatinib (Gleevec®)** was the first drug developed in this category. It specifically interferes with an enzyme called a *tyrosine kinase*. Many tyrosine kinases are present in the body, but chronic myelogenous leukemia and several other cancers have unique tyrosine kinases that are not present in normal cells. Because the growth of these cancers is driven by abnormal tyrosine kinases, they are perfect targets for targeted cancer therapy. Since the initial success of imatinib, other drugs that seek to inhibit tyrosine kinases have also been developed. Examples include nilotinib (Tasigna®) and dasatinib (Sprycel®).

- **Epidermal growth factor receptor (EGFR)** provides growth signals to normal cells *and* cancer cells. In several cancers, it can be overly active and promote cancer growth. Several drugs seek to inhibit EGFR, including gefitinib (Iressa®), erlotinib (Tarceva®), and lapatinib (Tykerb®). The EGFR can also be targeted using antibodies (see below).
- **Sunitinib (Sutent®) and sorafenib (Nexavar®)** are targeted agents that seek to disrupt the formation of blood vessels that feed cancer. They also have other anticancer properties.
- **Bortezomib (Velcade®)** inhibits the *proteosome*, a complex of enzymes that normally destroys proteins that are no longer needed. Inhibiting this function can be lethal to some cancer cells.
- **Histone deacetylase (HDAC)** enzymes are responsible for compacting the DNA, so that it is tightly wound and therefore assumes an inactive state. Some cancers use this and other methods to inactivate the DNA and turn off the genes that govern normal cell growth. Essentially, these cancers turn off the "brakes" that would slow uncontrolled cancer growth. *HDAC inhibitors* are drugs that seek to reactivate these dormant genes and turn the brakes back on. Vorinostat (Zolinza®) and romidepsin (Istodax®) are currently approved. There are many similar drugs in clinical trials—panobinostat (LBH589) is perhaps the most widely known.
- **mTOR (mammalian target of rapamycin)** regulates the growth and survival of some cancers. Temsirolimus (Toricel®) is an approved drug that targets mTOR, and similar drugs are in development.

As you can see from this partial list, many effective small-molecule targeted drugs have become a standard part of the resources available to medical practitioners. This work has mostly been completed in the last decade, and the field is growing rapidly. Expect more of these types of cancer drugs to emerge from laboratories and then be tested in clinical trials.

Monoclonal Antibodies

As discussed in Chapter 1, monoclonal antibodies designed to attack cancer targets are manufactured in pharmaceutical factories—rather than by stimulating the immune system to produce them. They have become important tools in the fight against cancer. In general, monoclonal antibodies work best when aimed at targets on the surface of the cell or in the circulation. Antibodies can be *naked*, meaning they are pure antibodies, or *conjugated*, meaning they are linked to a toxin or a radioactive molecule.

Examples of antibodies that target specific proteins on lymph or blood cells (lymphomas and leukemias) include alemtuzumab (Campath®), gemtuzumab ozogamicin (Mylotarg®), and rituximab (Rituxan®). Radiation-linked antibodies for cancers of the lymph nodes are ibritumomab (Zevalin®) and tositumomab (Bexxar®).

Cetuximab (Erbitux®) and panitumumab (Vectibix®) target the EGFR, which we discussed previously (see erlotinib). Trastuzumab (Herceptin®) targets another similar growth factor receptor that commonly occurs in breast cancer.

Bevacizumab (Avastin®) inhibits *vascular endothelial growth factor* (VEGF), a key regulator of blood vessel growth that supports the ability of cancers to grow and attract a blood supply.

Immunotherapy

There are a number of ways to stimulate immune cells to fight cancer. The oldest is by using *cytokines*, naturally occurring substances that promote inflammation in the body. For example, cytokines are responsible for the fever we often get when have the flu. Cytokines can be generated synthetically and given to individuals to activate their immune systems. The activation is not highly specific to cancer, but occasionally a more highly stimulated immune system can recognize that the abnormal cells of cancer are present and effectively attack them. IL-2 (Aldesleukin®), interferon (Intron-A®, Roferon-A®, and others), and granulocyte-macrophage colony stimulating factor (GM-CSF, Leukine®) are examples of cytokine cancer drugs currently in use.

There are a number of ways to stimulate immune cells to fight cancer. The oldest is by using cytokines, *naturally occurring substances that promote inflammation in the body. For example, cytokines are responsible for the fever we often get when have the flu.*

Cancer vaccines have also generated a lot of interest. They hold a lot of promise, but remain difficult to produce. With most infectious diseases, we immunize a person who has not yet been infected. This type of vaccine protects us against a foreign organism that can be readily recognized as an invader by the immune system. When dealing with cancer, we are fighting a disease that is already present, comes from within us, and has already been missed by the immune system. This makes the task much more difficult. Recently, sipuleucel-T (Provenge®) was the first cancer vaccine to show a survival difference and be approved for use. Many others are under investigation.

Monoclonal antibodies can also be used to stimulate the immune system. Like cytokines, this approach is not specific to cancer but provides a general stimulation of the immune system. The stimulation can be quite powerful and can result in both anticancer effects and side effects. Ipilumumab (Yervoy®) is the first such drug only recently approved. Others are being tested.

Differentiation Therapy

Some cancers, especially blood cancers (leukemias), closely resemble an uncontrolled accumulation of immature blood cells. These cells are unable to "grow up." The body needs mature cells to function properly, so it keeps sending signals to the bone marrow to make more. But because the cells are unable to mature, the immature cells accumulate in great numbers and overwhelm the bone marrow and eventually the whole body. There are situations in which the ability to mature can be restored, and cancerous cells can be rendered incapable of causing further harm. All trans-retinoic acid (ATRA, Vesanoid®) is an example of a differentiation therapy.

Gene Therapy

OGX-011 (custirsen) is an *antisense oligonucleotide* currently in phase III studies. It represents a class of drugs designed to silence specific genes. Although a number of attempts have been made to create drugs that work this way, so far, none has resulted in an approved drug. Nevertheless, this approach is appealing because we know quite a bit about which genes are active in cancers. The ability to silence these genes could lead to effective cancer treatments. Another strategy to silence genes is through the recently discovered RNA interference approach. Scientists unexpectedly discovered that tiny RNA molecules containing a short stretch of a gene's sequence are used in nature to shut down the genes. Drugs that use this approach are on the horizon.

Efforts are also being made to insert individual genes into the body to replace those that are defective. No specific drugs have yet emerged from this work.

A Last Word About Drugs

This partial listing is meant to give you some knowledge of the drugs and approaches that are being tested for the treatment of cancer. You may recognize some of the drugs mentioned, but it is unlikely you have encountered most of them. Literally hundreds of drugs are in early stage studies. Most belong, at least loosely, to the categories of drugs that we have described. Some are entirely new and will not have a cousin or fit into a category we have discussed in this chapter.

A well done and fairly comprehensive listing of currently available cancer drugs can be found at the National Cancer Institute's website: www.cancer.gov/cancertopics/druginfo/alphalist.

THE BOTTOM LINE

- Numerous drugs are used in the treatment of cancer.
- Chemotherapy remains the single largest category of cancer drugs.
- Targeted therapies are usually either small molecules or monoclonal antibodies. These therapies seek to exploit abnormalities specific to cancer cells.
- Immunologic therapies, which are treatments that stimulate the immune system, are beginning to emerge, with new drugs gaining approval after being proven effective in clinical trials.
- Gene-oriented therapies are still in their infancy but hold considerable promise.
- More work is needed, and many drugs are now in the testing stages.

10

The Future of Cancer Treatment and Clinical Trials: Personalized Medicine

A REVOLUTION IS COMING to cancer clinical trials and cancer therapy. Elements of this revolution are here now, and the future will bring many more. Many of the newest cancer drugs approved over the last decade represent a new generation of cancer treatments.

We all want to believe that our medical treatment is personal and tailored just for us, and it is—at least partly. Most cancer treatments, however, are still one-size-tries-to-fit-all. This is changing. Three research directions are likely to drive cancer research in the future: targeted therapy, personalized therapy, and pharmacogenomics.

TARGETED THERAPY

As discussed in Chapters 1 and 9, an increasing number of cancer drugs are designed to target specific defects that occur only in cancer cells and not in normal ones. This is how antibiotics are made, and their enormous success lies in the fact that they attack invading bacteria and not human tissue.

It has been far more difficult to find out what makes a human cancer cell different from the regular human cells from which it is derived.

Our understanding of this process is steadily increasing, and drugs are now being designed to exploit these newly discovered weaknesses of cancer. Imatinib mesylate (Gleevec®), discussed earlier, was one of the first such drugs to enter routine use. It has revolutionized the treatment of chronic myelogenous leukemia, as well as several other cancers. In August 2011, the U.S. Food and Drug Administration (FDA) approved vemurafenib (Zelboraf®) for the treatment of melanoma, the deadliest form of skin cancer. This drug targets *BRAF*—a protein that is abnormal in nearly half of melanomas and drives the cancer's growth. Vemurafenib will only be given to those patients whose cancer has the target mutation.

Targeted drugs have a good chance of being more effective and less toxic than most drugs currently in use. They also have a greater potential to be used in individualized therapy. Since these drugs have a specific target, it is possible to develop tests to determine whether that particular target is present in a specific individual.

Personalized Therapy

An increasing number of clinical trials ask participants to allow them to take a sample of their cancer cells as part of the research study. For cancers that circulate in the blood, such as leukemias, this may involve only a simple blood sample. For other types of cancer, a *biopsy* may be needed. Don't be surprised if you get such a request when you're contemplating a clinical trial. These tumor samples are used to better understand which cancers respond to which treatments. Fear of needles aside, this is a good and progressive step in conducting clinical trials, and it can provide benefits for everyone with cancer.

Modern biotechnology allows us to measure tens of thousands of characteristics in a single cancer sample! Such sophisticated *biologic signatures* may finally allow us to uncover some of the mysteries that underlie individual tumors.

It is likely that, in the near future, a sample of an individual's cancer will be carefully and extensively analyzed in the laboratory before any therapy is started. The results of this analysis will allow us to select a treatment that will likely work the first time, thereby avoiding lengthy and expensive treatments that are likely to have little or no positive effect in the patient. We are already seeing this approach with the newest melanoma treatment approved in 2011. When this vision is fully realized, cancer clinical trials and cancer therapy will look quite different than they do today. The enormous clinical trials that seek to measure benefit in large groups of patients may be replaced by smaller studies that focus on subgroups of patients whose cancers have specific treatable defects.

An even more exciting possibility is that, someday, we will begin moving away from cancer treatment chosen on the basis of where the cancer originated—such as the breast, prostate, lung, kidney, or colon—and instead treat cancers that have a specific defect for which we have a particularly effective drug. When this happens, cancer treatment will be far more effective and, as a result, much less treatment will be necessary. Patients will get the right treatment for their specific cancer from the beginning. We are not there yet, and the transformation will come gradually, but it will happen first in clinical trials.

Someday, we will begin moving away from cancer treatment chosen on the basis of where the cancer originated—such as the breast, prostate, lung, kidney, or colon—and instead treat cancers that have a specific defect for which we have a particularly effective drug.

In 2011, two new cancer treatments were approved that illustrate this new paradigm. Crizotinib (Xalkori®) was approved for the treatment of lung cancer that harbors a specific mutation in the ALK gene. Vemurafenib, mentioned above, became available for a specific type of melanoma. Both of these drugs produce much better results than conventional drugs, as long as the tumors contain the defect that the drug is designed to exploit. Both of these drugs were approved together with tests that will allow doctors to determine for each individual patient whether the drugs are right for them. We will see many more such drug–test combinations, and they promise to bring much better results to cancer patients. The approval of these two drugs shows that the era of personalized medicine has arrived.

Pharmacogenomics

As previously discussed, we cannot tell in advance who will benefit from which treatment, and we are equally unable to predict who will develop serious side effects and who will hardly even notice he is taking a new cancer drug. Matching drugs to cancers to improve results will require careful biologic analysis of the tumors. On the other hand, predicting and avoiding side effects will require a careful biologic analysis of the whole person.

The human genome, which cost several billion dollars to sequence initially, can now be sequenced in a few weeks for a few thousand dollars. Expensive yes, but not overwhelmingly so—and, in the near future, it will be possible to sequence a patient's genetic information for less than a thousand dollars in just a day or two. Maybe your health insurance will even pay for it—you can *always* hope!

Although our individual differences are not due solely to genetics, many of our differences and the things that make us unique are coded into our DNA. We expect that hidden somewhere within this code is the ability to predict how the body will react to various medications and treatments. In the future, we hope to be able to perform sophisticated laboratory tests that will enable us to predict which treatments will result in the greatest benefit and do the least harm to each individual patient—and at minimal cost. Let's hope this all happens sooner rather than later!

The Bottom Line

- Today's cancer care often uses a "one-size-fits-all" approach that does not work equally well for everyone.

- Even though we know that humanity is a collection of individuals, we have not been able to reliably predict who will or will not benefit from a particular cancer treatment, and who will or will not experience side effects.
- Cancer drugs that target defects occurring only in cancer cells—and not in normal cells—hold the promise of more effective, less toxic treatments. Several of these drugs are already available.
- Deep, comprehensive analysis of individual cancers may—and likely *will*—allow us to accurately predict which treatments are most likely to work for an individual.
- Comprehensive analyses of the genetic makeup of individuals may allow us to accurately predict who will, and who will not, suffer serious side effects.
- These new strategies will first be tested in clinical trials.
- You can expect that many future clinical trials will include sophisticated laboratory tests in addition to treatments. These tests will be designed to help select better treatments and identify the individuals who are most likely to benefit from a specific treatment.

A Final Word

YOU HAVE MADE IT TO THE END of the book—unless you read the last chapter first! We hope that reading it will send you off to face the world of clinical trials and challenging decisions with the key facts that will help you navigate the jungle of experimental therapy and make the decision to participate or not.

Tell Us What You Think

If you have tried to learn about the process of clinical trials, you have probably encountered a few misconceptions. We hope we have provided you with clear answers in this book. We are also available to answer your questions on our blog: www.cancer-clinical-trials.com. Please let us know about any questions that we have not answered, concerns that we have not addressed, or issues that we have not anticipated. We will do our best to respond online, so the entire community of cancer patients interested in clinical trials will have the information. Your input and suggestions will also help us to enrich and expand the next edition of this book through the feedback we get from you.

We wish you well in your journey. By choosing to read this book, you are taking charge of your cancer, becoming informed, and looking for options. Let this be just the beginning. You will find many sources of strength and support. Clinical trials and the experimental therapies they offer may be a part of your cancer treatment now or in the future, or you may decide not to participate. Ask questions, and never stop seeking the answers that you need to win the battle that you did not seek, but must now fight.

Glossary

Adjuvant A treatment designed to reduce the risk of cancer recurrence; given after the primary therapy. Most often, this is chemotherapy given after surgery. This kind of treatment is given when no visible cancer exists, but there is a chance that microscopic amounts of cancer have been left behind and could cause a recurrence without additional treatment.

Androgen deprivation therapy Treatment to suppress or block the production or action of male hormones. This is done by having the testicles removed, by taking female sex hormones, or by taking drugs that reduce the production of male hormones and/or block their action on cancer cells. Also called *androgen ablation* and *androgen suppression.* This treatment is used in prostate cancer. Also see *Hormonal therapy.*

Antibody A blood protein, made by B cells (white blood cells) and designed to attach to a specific antigen. One of the main parts of the immune system.

Benign Not malignant or cancerous.

Biologic agents A broad definition of cancer drugs that seek to manipulate a specific target in the cancer to treat it. Biologic agents include antibodies, small molecules, and immune therapies.

Biologically effective dose A dose high enough to have the desired effect on cancer cells. A dose that successfully hits the target.

Biopsy A procedure that takes a small sample of tissue (specimen) from a tumor. A biopsy is commonly obtained using a relatively thick needle that is inserted into the tumor, often using ultrasound or a computed tomography (CT) scan to guide the needle. A biopsy can also be done surgically.

Blinded studies Studies or clinical trials that utilize placebos or other means to assign patients to different treatments in such a way that the patient, and usually the doctor, do not know which treatment is being administered. A method to reduce biases in research results.

Blood counts Actual counting of key subtypes of blood cells in the blood. Primarily counts of white cells (immune cells that can be reduced dramatically with chemotherapy), red cells (the main part of the blood; the oxygen carrying cells; low red cells means anemia), and platelets (cells responsible for blood clotting).

Blood chemistries Blood tests that measure electrolytes—such things as calcium, sodium, potassium, and sugar (glucose)—as well as substances that estimate kidney and liver function. Also known as a *chemistry panel.* Various chemistry panels measure a smaller or a larger number of substances; they can range from six or seven (basic panel), to as many as 20 (complete or comprehensive panel).

Bone marrow Located in the center of bones, the source of all blood cells.

Bone scan Also known as *bone scintigraphy.* A technique that creates images of bones on a computer screen or on film. A small amount of radioactive material is injected into a blood vessel and then travels through the bloodstream; it collects in the bones and is detected by a scanner. Bone scan abnormalities can reflect cancer in the bones, but could also be due to benign causes such as arthritis, fracture, inflammation, or bone injury.

Breast cancer Cancer that forms in tissues of the breast, usually the ducts (tubes that carry milk to the nipple) and lobules (glands that make milk). It occurs in both men and women, although male breast cancer is rare.

Cancer Also known as *neoplasm.* A disease of abnormal, uncontrolled cell growth that leads to invasion of nearby tissues and spreads to other parts of the body through the blood and lymph systems. Cancers are always named after the organ or part of their body in which they originated. There are many types of cancer.

Cancer-free No identifiable cancer cells in the body. Also known as *in remission.* This is not the same as being cured. Sometimes microscopic, invisible amounts of cancer can remain and cause the cancer to come back. See *Relapse.*

Cancer staging Performing exams and tests to learn the extent of the cancer within the body, especially whether the disease has spread from the original site to other parts of the body. It is important to know the stage of the disease in order to plan the best treatment. Staging typically involves a physical examination and scans or X-rays. The exact types of scans ordered depend on the type of cancer. For some cancers, full staging also involves blood tests. *Clinical staging* means that the cancer stage was determined purely using examination, scans, and perhaps blood tests. *Pathologic staging* means that surgery for cancer was performed, and the size and extent of the cancer was in part evaluated by looking at the tumor and surrounding tissue that was removed. The two staging approaches are not equivalent; pathologic staging is more invasive, but also more accurate.

Cancer survivor A person who has or has had cancer and is alive. Often thought of as a person who has completed initial treatment for his or her cancer.

Chemotherapy The treatment of disease using chemicals that have a specific toxic effect upon the disease-producing microorganisms (antibiotics) or that selectively destroy cancerous tissue (anticancer therapy).

Clinical trial An experiment in which new drugs, combinations of drugs, other treatments, or medical devices are tested in human volunteers. Tends to be highly organized and regimented with respect to qualification to participate, as well as to all procedures. Sometimes referred to as a *clinical study* or just *study*, although these terms have a broader meaning.

Clinical study Includes clinical trials in which an active intervention is tested, as well as noninterventional studies, such as those that collect information about people to better understand causes of disease or associations between risk factors and diseases. All clinical trials are clinical studies, but some clinical studies—those that are not testing an intervention—are not clinical trials.

Colorectal cancer A malignancy that arises from the lining of either the colon or the rectum. Cancers of the large intestine are the second most common form of cancer found in men and women.

Crossover An element of study design that allows patients to receive one of two treatments first and the other treatment later.

Contraindication A condition or factor that increases the risks involved in using a particular drug, carrying out a medical procedure, or engaging in a particular activity. A *relative contraindication* indicates that, although the risks are increased, the treatment or procedure might still be prudently carried out. An *absolute contraindication* means that the treatment or procedure cannot be carried out safely and should not be done.

CT scan Also known as a CAT scan. CT stands for *computed tomography.* A special radiographic technique that uses a computer to assemble multiple X-ray images into a two-dimensional cross-sectional image.

Cyst A closed sac having a distinct membrane and separation from the nearby tissue. It may contain air, fluids, or semi-solid material. Once formed, a cyst may go away by itself, or it may have to be removed surgically. Cysts can sometimes become cancerous, but they are most often benign.

Diagnosis The process of identifying a disease, such as cancer. Typically involves multiple tests. Cancer is definitively diagnosed by examining a sample of tissue (see *Biopsy*) under a microscope.

DNA Deoxyribonucleic acid; the material that carries our genetic code. Located in the nucleus of nearly all cells of the human body.

Double-blinding See *Blinded studies.* A study design element that calls for neither the patient nor his or her doctor to know which of two or more treatments is being prescribed in a study. A method to reduce bias in clinical trial results.

DSMB A data safety monitoring board (sometimes also called a committee) is an independent group responsible for reviewing the results of clinical trials while they are active. Most of the time, they are responsible for larger randomized trials in which the DSMB has the responsibility to stop a study if one of the treatments proves clearly superior or clearly inferior to the other.

Eligibility Meeting the requirements (such as disease type or stage, health status, or age range) in order to participate in a clinical trial. Eligibility criteria typically involve an extensive list of *inclusion criteria*—things you must have to participate, and *exclusion criteria*—things that would exclude a person from participation. All criteria must be satisfied to qualify for a clinical trial. A *checklist* is often used to facilitate the eligibility review process.

Enzyme A chemical that serves as a catalyst for a specific chemical reaction. Cells in our bodies use enzymes to make specific chemicals.

Equipoise A requirement for randomized studies. Agreement that all treatment choices available through a study are equally valid and that we do not know with confidence that one is superior to another.

Estrogen One of a group of compounds that are the primary female sex hormones. Estrogen promote the growth of certain forms of breast cancer, which indicates that the cancer may be responsive to hormonal treatments.

Experiment A procedure designed to test a hypothesis. An experiment proves a hypothesis to be true or shows it to be false. This is a core element in the scientific process of searching for knowledge.

Experimental medicine A broad term that defines any medical care activity that is not standard and is being investigated in a systematic and organized fashion. Clinical trials are an example of experimental medicine.

Experimental drug Also referred to as an *investigational drug.* A medication that is not currently approved for routine use by the U.S. Food and Drug Administration (FDA) and is being evaluated in clinical trials.

External beam radiation A therapy that uses high-energy rays or particles to destroy cancer cells or slow their rate of growth. A carefully focused beam of radiation is delivered from a machine outside the body.

FDA U.S. Food and Drug Administration. The federal agency that regulates, among other things, medications and medical devices.

FDA approval A requirement for a drug to be sold in the United States. The FDA only approves drugs that are safe and effective. Meeting this standard can require large, complex studies and an extensive review process.

Gene therapy This cancer treatment, which is largely still experimental, seeks to insert healthy genes into cancers that are caused or driven by faulty genes. A related strategy involves turning off genes in cancer cells that are inappropriately turned on and actively contributing to the cancer process.

Gold standard The best standard treatment currently available.

Growth signal A biologic message that tells cells to grow. The message is typically conveyed through a chemical, such as a hormone. The human body sends many signals to different body parts to coordinate their functioning.

Hormonal therapy Treatment that adds, blocks, or removes hormones. Synthetic hormones, hormone blockers, or other drugs may be given to block the body's natural hormones in order to slow or stop the growth of certain tumors, such as prostate cancer and breast cancer.

Hormone A chemical that circulates in the blood and regulates the behavior of specific cells in the body. Hormones are made in one gland, but can affect cells all over the body. Examples of hormones include testosterone and estrogen but there are many others. Some cancers, such as breast and prostate cancer, may be fueled by hormones.

Hypothesis A tentative proposal or an idea that needs to be tested in an experiment to determine whether it is correct. Every experiment, including a clinical trial, begins with a hypothesis and then seeks to prove it or disprove it. The hypothesis is a cornerstone of the scientific process.

Imaging The general field of using various technologies to get a picture of an area inside the body. Commonly used techniques include ultrasound, X-ray, computed tomography (CT) scan, magnetic resonance imaging (MRI), positron emission tomography (PET) scan, and nuclear medicine scans.

Immunotherapy A treatment that seeks to mobilize the immune system to fight cancer. There are many different ways to do this. A few treatments have been approved and entered into routine use. Many more are being studied.

Informed consent The process of informing a potential study participant of the particulars of the study, especially its potential risks, benefits, and alternative strategies, as well as the participant's rights and responsibilities. A study volunteer can indicate his or her consent to participate by signing a consent form, but only after having a solid understanding of all of these issues. This is required for participation in a clinical trial.

Investigational agent A drug that has not been approved by the FDA, but that has been approved for testing in humans in clinical trials.

IV Intravenous. An injection or infusion (drip) directly into the vein. Used for drugs that cannot be absorbed by mouth. Typically, a soft plastic catheter (tube) is inserted into a vein using a sharp needle. Once placed, the needle is removed and the drug, fluids, or blood are given through the catheter.

Laparoscopic surgery Surgery performed using instruments that allow surgeons to see and operate inside the human body using only small incisions. Surgery using tools that are similar to periscopes.

Leukemia Cancer of the bone marrow. Manifests itself through aggressive overgrowth of white blood cells. A number of subtypes of leukemia are defined by the type of white cells involved.

Lumpectomy The surgical removal of a lump (usually a tumor or cancer lump) without the removal of the entire organ. The term is most often used to describe surgery for breast cancer.

Lung cancer Cancer that forms in tissues of the lung, usually in the cells lining air passages.

Lymph nodes Organs consisting of many types of cells; they are a part of the lymphatic system. Lymph nodes are found throughout the body, and they act as filters or traps for foreign particles. Lymph nodes contain white blood cells. They are important in the proper functioning of the immune system. Many cancers can spread to lymph nodes, forming metastases.

Metastases Tumors formed by a cancer that has spread from its organ of origin to distant locations. This type of cancer is known as *metastatic.* The patterns of spread vary among cancers. Common sites include lymph nodes, lungs, bones, and the liver, but metastases can involve any organ of the body.

Malignant Cancerous. Malignant tumors can invade and destroy nearby tissue and spread to other parts of the body.

Mastectomy The surgical removal of the entire breast. Also see *Lumpectomy.*

Medicaid The federal and state health insurance program for low-income individuals and families.

Medicare The federal health insurance program for those over the age of 65.

MRI Magnetic resonance imaging; an imaging procedure that uses powerful magnetic energy linked to a computer to create detailed pictures of areas inside the body. These pictures can show the difference between normal and diseased tissue.

MTD Maximum tolerated dose; refers to the highest dose of a drug that is reasonably safe for patients to take. This does *not* mean free of side effects, but rather that the level of side effects is thought to be acceptable in a specific situation. A drug that has a chance of curing an otherwise lethal cancer may be given even with considerable side effects. This is as contrasted with, for example, a drug used to treat high blood pressure for a lifetime, which needs to be safe and have minimal side effects.

Mutation A defect in the genetic code (also see *DNA*) that often leads to an abnormal protein. Many cancers are caused by mutations in the DNA. Mutations can also occur in healthy cells without causing cancer. The nature of each mutation determines its effect on health and disease.

NCI National Cancer Institute. The principal federal institution dedicated to advancing cancer care through research. The most important and largest single source of funding for cancer research.

Oncologist A physician who specializes in treating cancer. Medical oncologists focus on the use of medications to treat cancers and often see patients with more advanced cancers. A *surgical oncologist* is a surgeon with special training and expertise in cancer surgery. A *radiation oncologist* is trained in the use of radiation to treat cancer.

Oncology The study and treatment of cancer.

Personalized medicine Medical care built on the principle that individuals respond differently and uniquely to treatments, and that treatments should be selected for each person based on an understanding of the unique biology both of his disease and his body. Personalized medicine is gradually becoming a reality, but in many conditions it remains a goal that requires further research before it can be fully realized.

PET scan Positron emission tomography. An imaging modality that uses a variety of *contrast agents* (given by IV) to generate pictures inside the body that reflect function, such as metabolic activity. This differs from other types of imaging, which focus on structure rather than function. PET has advantages in imaging of certain cancers that may have higher metabolic activity than normal healthy tissues.

PET-CT A combination scan that includes both positron emission tomography (PET) and computed tomography (CT), with the pictures fused to create one set of images. This approach combines imaging structures with an analysis of their function.

Placebo An inactive substance or treatment that looks the same as, and is given in the same way as, an active drug or treatment being tested. The effects of the active drug or treatment are compared to the effects of the placebo.

Pharma An abbreviation for "pharmaceutical." Often used to refer to a pharmaceutical company or the entire pharmaceutical industry.

PK Pharmacokinetics. The study of drug levels in the body of the patient and how they change over time as drugs are absorbed, distributed, metabolized, and excreted.

Placebo effect Getting better as the result of treatments other than an active medication.

Progesterone A hormone involved in the female menstrual cycle, reproduction, and pregnancy. Progesterone promotes the growth of certain forms of breast cancer, which indicates that the cancer may be responsive to hormonal treatments.

Prognosis The likely outcome or course of a disease; the chance of recovery or recurrence. Typically based on knowledge from studies of many patients. It is important to know that a prognosis is an educated guess using what we know happens on average in order to estimate the chances of something happening in the future. We don't know for sure what will actually happen with a single individual.

Prostate cancer Cancer that forms in the tissues of the prostate (a gland in the male reproductive system found below the bladder and in front of the rectum).

Proton beam radiation A novel form of radiation therapy that relies on bombarding cancer with protons, the tiny positively charged molecules found in the nuclei of atoms of all elements.

Radiation Energy released in the form of particle or electromagnetic waves, such as medical X-rays.

Random assignment Assigning or allocating patients to different treatments in a random way, usually by computer. The most objective means for reducing bias in the composition of the experimental and control groups. A trial with random assignment is termed a *randomized-controlled* clinical trial, or more simply, a randomized trial.

Relapse Also known as *recurrence*; the cancer comes back after treatment.

Screening Tests done to detect cancer early in individuals who feel and appear healthy, and who show no visible evidence of cancer.

Side effects Unintended negative effects of medications or treatments. Also known as *adverse events.*

Signed informed consent A signed document required for participation in a clinical trial. See *Informed consent.*

Standard treatment The best treatment currently approved by the FDA and in routine use.

Sugar pill A placebo or neutral treatment.

Surgery Cutting into the human body for medical purposes.

Survival benefit The life-prolonging effect of a treatment.

Targeted therapy Treatments that seek to use drugs to attack specific weak points in cancer that are vulnerable to attack. Targeted therapy requires the ability to identify the correct targets and the ability to make drugs that are specific and only affect their targets while leaving the rest of the body alone.

Testosterone The male sex hormone.

Therapeutic intent The determination that an experimental treatment has a goal of making the patient better, as distinct from a purely scientific goal, such as the measurement of drug levels.

Trial phases Clinical trials are conducted in a series of steps, called *phases*—each phase is designed to answer a separate research question.

Tumor An abnormal mass of tissue that results when cells divide more than they should or do not die when they should. Tumors may be *benign* (not cancerous) or *malignant* (cancerous).

Tumor markers Substances made by tumors that can be measured in blood samples; they can be used to roughly estimate the status of the cancer. These are different for different cancers (and don't exist for some). Examples include PSA in prostate cancer, CA-125 in ovarian cancer, and CEA in colorectal cancer.

Urologist A physician who specializes in diseases of the urinary organs in women and the urinary and sex organs in men. Urologic oncologists have special training in the surgical management of cancers of the prostate, bladder, kidneys, and testicles.

Resources

General Clinical Trials Information

We recommend starting your search for information about clinical trials using these more general comprehensive websites. Internet links often change, but if a link doesn't work for you, simply type the name of the organization into a search engine such as Google to get a current address.

The authors of this book also will be pleased to respond to your questions on their blog at: www.cancer-clinical-trials.com. You can also contact them on Facebook at: facebook.com/CancerClinicalTrials.

- **www.cancer.gov** The National Cancer Institute's website containing comprehensive information about every kind of cancer and cancer treatment, as well as clinical trials.
- **www.cancer.gov/clinicaltrials** The National Cancer Institute's subpage devoted to clinical trials. Location of the most important search engine for finding clinical trials.
- **www.cancer.org** The American Cancer Society's website. The most comprehensive nongovernmental source of information about cancer and its treatment.
- **www.cancer.org/treatment/treatmentsandsideeffects/clinicaltrials/app/clinical-trials-matching-service.aspx** The American Cancer Society's clinical trials matching service.
- **www.ncbi.nlm.nih.gov/pubmed** The National Library of Medicine's PubMed service. This is a comprehensive search engine for medical publications. At least the abstract, and sometimes the entire text of nearly all scientific publications related to medicine, can be located here.

- **www.cancer.net/patient/All+About+Cancer/Clinical+Trials** The American Society of Clinical Oncology website containing information about cancer clinical trials.
- **www.clinicaltrials.gov** The National Institute of Health search engine for clinical trials. This website allows you to search for clinical trials for all conditions. You might want to start with the National Cancer Institute's search site, which is focused on cancer, but you may also encounter this site in your searches.
- **www.cancertrialshelp.org** Cancer trials information from the national cooperative groups. These are the largest federally supported groups conducting large-scale trials in the United States.
- **www.centerwatch.com** A comprehensive website devoted to industry-sponsored clinical trials.
- **www.acor.org/clinical.html** Association of Cancer Online Resources is a comprehensive offering of online peer support groups and patient-centered web sites. Some of the offerings include information about clinical trials.

Many resources are devoted to specific types of cancer. If your cancer is not among the most common, you will probably find similar resources online by typing in *clinical trials information for the cancer of interest* into a general search engine window.

Information Specific by Tumor Type

These selected resources are specific for the most common cancers and offer additional information:

- Lung Cancer
  Lung Cancer Alliance: www.lungcanceralliance.org/facing/trials.html
- Prostate Cancer
  Prostate Cancer Foundation: www.pcf.org
- Colorectal Cancer
  Fight Colorectal Cancer: www.fightcolorectalcancer.org
- Breast Cancer
  BreastCancerTrials.org: www.breastcancertrials.org
  Susan G. Komen for the Cure Foundation: www.komen.org

Index

Note: Boldface numbers indicate illustrations; italic t indicates a table.